YOGA
FOR
CANCER

"*Yoga for Cancer* is a look into Tari's simple yet groundbreaking work with survivors. Her practical guide helps cancer survivors create a safe and inspiring home yoga practice. Tari's gentle approach is complemented perfectly by her easy-to-follow guidance, making *Yoga for Cancer* an instrumental aspect of healing, surviving, and thriving after treatment.

ELENA BROWER, COAUTHOR OF *ART OF ATTENTION*

"As a general oncologist, I wholeheartedly support *Yoga for Cancer*. Tari has successfully blended the ancient art of yoga with the contemporary art of oncology in a beautifully mindful but scientifically based manner."

JULIE J. OLIN, M.D., MEDICAL ONCOLOGY,
FLETCHER ALLEN HEALTH CARE, VERMONT

"*Yoga for Cancer* is a yoga prescription for those touched by cancer. Tari offers support born of experience and tough love liberally sprinkled with compassion. As a writer and yoga teacher, I can say this book makes an important contribution to our collective knowledge of the healing powers of yoga."

LINDA SPARROWE, AUTHOR OF *YOGA—A YOGA JOURNAL BOOK* AND
FORMER MANAGING EDITOR OF *YOGA JOURNAL*

"*Yoga for Cancer* is a must read for all those living with cancer, providing the essential yoga tools with which you can construct your own wellness plan. If you are living with cancer and have tried yoga before or need an invitation to start, please read this book."

KATE MCINTYRE CLERE, WRITER, DIRECTOR, FILMMAKER FOR *YOGAWOMAN*

"*Yoga for Cancer* is a wonderful read and full of essential information for those living with breast cancer."

LINDA AND BOB CAREY, FOUNDERS OF THE TUTU PROJECT

"Tari's empathy and knowledge of how the body works is a tremendous benefit to all who read *Yoga for Cancer*."

MIO FREDLAND, M.D., PSYCHIATRIST, NEW YORK
PRESBYTERIAN UNIVERSITY HOSPITAL OF COLUMBIA AND CORNELL

"A wonderful aid for beginners like me."

"Tari's passion to assist cancer survivors is outstanding. Her practice is easy to follow and helps us get over the past and move more powerfully in the future. She provides mind and body empowerment."

"Tari Prinster was my Yoda-in-a-tank-top. I began taking her yoga classes simply to get back the range of motion in my arm and chest muscles, but her class taught me much more. I left stronger, inside and out. She expresses the lessons of her classes now in this book, and I'm thrilled she'll get to touch so many more people."

"*Yoga for Cancer* is a fact-based guide to healing. Tari explains in clear language *what* to do and *why* to unlock the healing potential of yoga."

"While I was going through cancer treatments a few years ago, Tari's classes really helped me focus on something else besides being sick. The techniques and wisdom in *Yoga for Cancer* are almost as good as having Tari right there with you."

"This book is a terrific guide for survivors to do a daily practice. Its goal is to make this method of yoga for cancer a beacon for every survivor in the form of a book. Tari did a wonderful job creating this step-by-step method, and survivors everywhere will benefit."

"As a cancer survivor myself, I found Tari's information on how to detoxify our body to be invaluable to my recovery. *Yoga for Cancer* is a useful tool for helping cancer survivors to reclaim their lives."

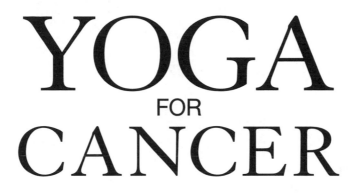

YOGA
FOR
CANCER

A Guide to Managing
Side Effects, Boosting Immunity,
and Improving Recovery
for Cancer Survivors

TARI PRINSTER

Healing Arts Press
Rochester, Vermont • Toronto, Canada

Healing Arts Press
One Park Street
Rochester, Vermont 05767
www.HealingArtsPress.com

Healing Arts Press is a division of Inner Traditions International

Note to the reader: This book is intended as an informational guide. The remedies, approaches, and techniques described herein are meant to supplement, and not to be a substitute for, professional medical care or treatment. They should not be used to treat a serious ailment without prior consultation with a qualified health care professional.

Library of Congress Cataloging-in-Publication Data
Prinster, Tari, 1944– author.
  Yoga for cancer : a guide to managing side effects, boosting immunity, and improving recovery for cancer survivors / Tari Prinster.
    pages cm
  Includes bibliographical references and index.
  ISBN 978-1-62055-272-8 (pbk.) — ISBN 978-1-62055-273-5 (e-book)
  1. Cancer—Exercise therapy. 2. Hatha yoga—Therapeutic use. 3. Cancer—Patients—Rehabilitation. I. Title.
  RC271.Y63P75 2014
  616.99'4062—dc23

                                                                        2014005465

Printed and bound in the United States by P. A. Hutchison

10 9 8 7 6 5 4 3 2 1

Text design by Priscilla Baker and layout by Debbie Glogover
This book was typeset in Garamond Premier Pro with Gill Sans MT Pro, Helvetica Neue LT Std, and ITC Legacy Sans Std display fonts

To send correspondence to the author of this book, mail a first-class letter to the author c/o Inner Traditions • Bear & Company, One Park Street, Rochester, VT 05767, and we will forward the communication, or contact the author directly at **www.y4c.com**.

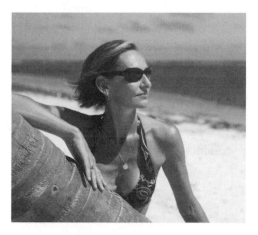

This book is dedicated to the late
Kelly Considine (March 17, 1965–January 11, 2013),
my able assistant and friend.
She fearlessly confronted her cancer for seven years.
Until her last breath, she used her yoga practice
to make sense of and ease her suffering.
These words express her wisdom and great courage.

*A strong yet gentle practice is how I am surviving. When asked
by the doctors how I support my spine, I tell them, "with my
core." If that were weak, my back would break. Aside from the
strength, yoga keeps me focused. It allows me to flow and breathe
and stretch out all the sadness, the fear, and the anxiety. I see it,
I flow with it, and I let it go.*

KELLY CONSIDINE

AUTHOR'S NOTE

Throughout this book you will read vignettes written by some of my yoga students, yoga teachers I have trained, and yoga friends who have been touched by or are living with cancer. These brief narratives are written about their personal experience of recovery using yoga. There has been minimal editing of their words to protect personal identity.

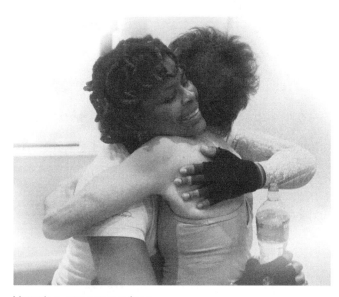

Veronica, cancer survivor

Contents

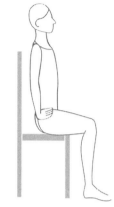

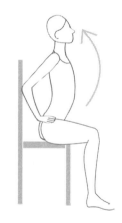

PART 1

Understanding Cancer and the Benefits of Yoga

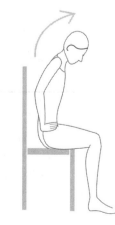

PART 2

How to Build Your Own Yoga Practice

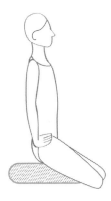

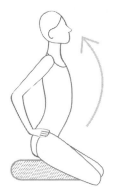

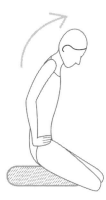

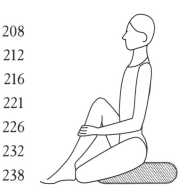
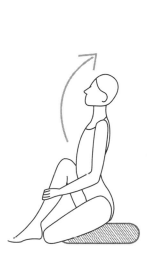
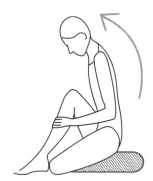

Foreword

Cyndi Lee, founder of OM yoga

The first time I met Tari Prinster was at OM yoga, my yoga studio in New York City. Along with forty-nine other people, Tari was attending an informational meeting about the upcoming OM yoga teacher training program I was offering. After explaining the nuts and bolts of the program I invited questions, and Tari's hand went up. "Do you have to be able to do a pose in order to teach it?"

Good question, and a fairly typical one. But Tari was not typical. My Greenwich Village yoga studio was full of strong and hyper-agile dancers in their twenties and thirties. Tari looked to be in her midfifties, a rare demographic for urban yoga studios in 2000, and that fact alone distinguished her as someone curious and confident, maybe even courageous. I wondered what it was she thought she couldn't do. As I looked at her more closely, I wondered what she would do, because it was clear that she could probably do whatever she wanted. Despite learning of her hip injury, I readily accepted her into the program.

Flash forward ten years to the Forest studio at OM yoga, where, along with twenty other women, I am wrapped in duct tape. This was one of Tari's brilliant ideas for helping the participants in our OM yoga Woman Cancer Survivor Teacher Training course understand the physical restrictions that often result from breast cancer treatments and surgeries. We pulled the tape tight around our abdomens to feel what it would be like to have our belly fat removed to make a new breast. We used it to strap down our upper arms, disabling lifting movements as if we'd had lymph nodes removed.

The duct tape made us laugh at first, but then people became deeply emotional and the tears flowed. Tari understood that emulating cancer's potential physical restrictions was just a gateway to helping us feel, in our breath, bones, muscles, and heart, the experiences of those whom we were trying to help.

Through her years of dedication to this work, Tari had found the answer to her original question, with a variation: "Do you have to have cancer to teach yoga to cancer survivors?" No, but it helps if you can somehow embody what it feels like to walk the path of a cancer survivor.

What happened in the years between her question and her answer is the story of the OM yoga Woman Cancer Survivor program, the development of y4c (yoga4cancer), and how Tari's "ministry" became a book.

The OM yoga Woman Cancer Survivor program began when I got a call from the Libby Ross Foundation, looking for a place to hold cancer survivor yoga classes. This was a welcome request, because our mission included a commitment to 1) teach the best yoga possible to as many people as possible and 2) create community. Libby Ross Foundation's request fit this perfectly. And we embraced the opportunity wholeheartedly.

One of the best communal aspects of OM yoga was, of course, the women's dressing room! Great conversations, news, ideas, connections—it all happened there. One day on my way to change, Tari mentioned that she'd heard we needed a new teacher for the Yoga for Cancer class. She was right. The teacher was getting married soon and moving on. Tari politely mentioned that she would really like to teach the class if I thought that would work. I thought about it for maybe two seconds and said, "Yes! That is the perfect solution!" I knew that Tari had had breast cancer and that she would be able to relate to the students. What I didn't know was that this opportunity was the beginning of Tari's ministry. I didn't know that she would take all the structures, guidelines, and philosophies that she had learned at OM and modify them to create a new way of teaching yoga that was precisely designed to help women with cancer.

The mantra of a good yoga teacher is "How can I be helpful?" Through diligent study and determined practice, a good teacher is well prepared to personally connect with and help anyone who walks into her classroom.

And that has been Tari's true gift to women cancer survivors: a way of teaching yoga that helps them reconnect with themselves. With a cancer diagnosis, many women have lost their hair and bone density, the ability to balance life and hold down a job, and maybe even their life partner. The fear and sadness can be overwhelming. It's not easy to look at one's body after disfiguring surgery. It's not easy to face the day with a broken heart.

Being shown that you can still experience strength, sanity, and your own basic goodness is huge. Being gently guided toward renewing a healthy, positive, and loving relationship with one's own body—a body that has or once had cancer—is also huge. And Tari brought those offerings to her classes at the OM yoga center for eight years—and continues indefatigably to do so throughout New York City.

Tari hasn't stopped her ministry to write this book. She is teaching every day and continuing to help every single person who walks into her classroom. With this book, even more people will reap the benefits of her insights, research, experience, and unfailing generosity. I am honored to have helped Tari find her path and proud of how she's made it her own. May her generosity, knowledge, and compassion continue to serve the women who need her most.

CYNDI LEE is the first female Western yoga teacher to fully integrate yoga asana and Tibetan Buddhism into her practice and teaching. Founder of NYC's influential OM yoga, Cyndi now teaches workshops and teacher trainings worldwide. Author of the yoga classic *Yoga Body Buddha Mind*, her newest book is *May I Be Happy: A Memoir of Love, Yoga and Changing My Mind*. www.cyndilee.com

Foreword

Robyn Frankel-Tiger, M.D.

As a physician, I spent fifteen years in diagnostic radiology. I was the face that patients saw when they came for their mammograms, ultrasounds, and biopsies. I was the face they saw when they were told they had cancer. I was the face they saw each time they came back for the results of their radiology studies following their biopsies, surgeries, chemotherapy, and radiation, holding on tightly to the hands of loved ones, hoping to receive good news.

This is what *I* repeatedly saw: the innumerable faces of women filled with emotional anguish and dampened spirits hopelessly associated with their debilitating physical bodies. I knew that my job as a doctor was not nearly complete. What more could I do? Beyond giving a hug and a smile, I was completely lost as to how to help these women heal.

What I did know was that the one thing that continually helped me heal from life's noncancerous physical and emotional challenges was my yoga practice. My scientifically trained mind needed to unwrap the mystifying impact of yoga at a deeper, fact-based level. I originally studied to be a yoga teacher to deepen my own practice and understanding of the human body and mind. It was through my studies that I was introduced to the field of yoga therapy and began studying with the organization Integrative Yoga Therapy. During that training I learned that medical research has proved that yoga lessens the side effects of cancer therapies during and after treatment.

This newfound knowledge ignited a brightly glowing light in my mind and a passion in my heart. It was imperative that I learn more. As the saying goes, "When the student is ready, the teacher will appear." When I first met Tari Prinster, I knew I had found the perfect teacher.

Studying with Tari was life changing. She taught me that true compassion is attained in two ways: first through knowledge, and then through understanding. Her methodology was a combination of her personal experience, knowledge of human physiology, understanding of cancer and its treatments, and her expertise in yoga. As a physician, I respected her foundation in science. It was clear this knowledge is required to work effectively with those affected by cancer.

I will never forget how she brought me to understand a cancer survivor's pain and challenges. In the experiential portion of the training, my classmates and I were instructed to create the physical limitations of a cancer survivor with the aid of props to our own bodies. Once padded and restricted, we participated in a full yoga class. Tari is right in saying, "Cancer steals your breath; yoga gives it back." Toward the beginning of class, while physically restrained and full of emotion, I actually felt that I could not breathe. My body was failing me. Responsively, yoga brought back my breath. This was one of the most moving and humbling experiences of my life. It helped me understand the challenges survivors face.

Tari's passion to help other survivors extends outside the yoga studio. In this book, *Yoga for Cancer,* Tari masterfully describes in detail how to create a safe and effective yoga practice and also provides the reader with the facts on why one should use yoga to improve her or his quality of life. It is well written, informative, and has clear and easy-to-follow instructions. *Yoga for Cancer* gives clear explanation of the science behind cancer and how yoga can strengthen the immune system. For these reasons it is an excellent resource for my yoga therapy and medical colleagues. Most importantly, *Yoga for Cancer* is an invaluable tool for allowing survivors to take an active and important role in their own healing process. It should be part of every patient's recovery program.

I am forever grateful for Tari as I now have two additional ways to help my patients heal. First, her creative teachings have given me the ability to touch the lives of so many people through yoga therapy. Second, when those emotionally anguished faces stare at me for guidance, I will hand them this book along with a hug and a smile. Thank you, Tari!

Namaste!

Robyn Frankel-Tiger, M.D., founder of Yoga Heals 4 Life, is a physician and yoga therapist in southern New Jersey. Her therapeutic yoga practice integrates traditional Western medicine with the Eastern science of yoga. Her passion for helping those living with cancer grew out of her many years in medical practice witnessing firsthand the need for more complete patient care. Ultimately, her vision is the inclusion of therapeutic yoga for cancer as part of every patient's treatment plan, giving each patient the opportunity to take an active role in his or her journey to healing.

Preface

A cancer diagnosis changes your life in an instant. No matter the diagnosis or prognosis, fear, regret, and bewilderment take over. You feel a complete loss of power and control over your body, emotions, and life. Your cancer team—from family to doctors to supporters—lovingly help you manage your disease, your treatments, your life, and your well-being. Throughout your journey, whether it is short or lifelong, you have procedures done to you, advice provided, and love given.

All that is great, but if you are like me, you feel like you lose your independence. Surgeries take parts of your body. Treatments take away your clarity of mind and energy. Your medical team makes many decisions for you. Fear threatens to take it all from you. You feel powerless, lost in uncertainty. Your hope is to be "normal" again, to have the physical and emotional strength to do what once came naturally and easily. You want to feel a sense of control, stability, and hope.

For me yoga became my companion on a long journey, my ally to encourage me to take an *active* role in my recovery. It empowered me to be healthier and stronger than I ever was before the cancer. Most importantly, it provided me the time and support for self-awareness and self-love. In fact, it enabled me to build, I hope, a better version of myself, a person dedicated to helping others find power, love, and support through yoga.

I was, and remain, a skeptic about broad promises that often come with yoga or many cancer treatments. I respect Eastern philosophy and ancient traditions, but am not a follower or convert. I am too pragmatic.

Impermanence is our home and loss the law of the world.

Pico Iyer

The development of my yoga practice was driven by curiosity, insight, research, and applied practice with the hundreds of survivors with whom I have personally worked. My approach—y4c (yoga4cancer) methodology—as described in the book, is based on fact-based science and research. My approach is about improving your odds, giving your body the tools to fight harder and more effectively during active treatment or in the years after. I want to share what I have learned.

Know this: questions and a fighting spirit are more important than the facts, which change as we learn more about how cancer can be managed and about the way yoga supports wellness. Being curious, asking questions, demanding answers, but also learning patience—this approach helps us take back our lives. This is what I care about most.

I want this book to be useful to everyone touched by and living with cancer, whatever stage and whatever phase of the cancer journey. Caregivers and health care professionals can also benefit from understanding more about yoga and its use in managing cancer and the side effects of treatment.

Also, I hope that this book helps compassionate yoga teachers become more aware of the cancer community and their needs for healing. I often say to my teachers in training that "true compassion flows from understanding and facts." So another aim of this book is that the research and the rationale behind the choice of poses presented here will help more yoga teachers help more survivors to live longer, healthier, and happier lives.

Writing a book, especially if one is not a natural writer, is a huge project! Over five years my book changed shape so many times. What you are reading now represents the thinking and countless hours of editing of many people whom I wish to thank. The first thank you goes to my own students, who cannot be acknowledged by name—students in yoga classes, yoga teacher trainings, and yoga retreats—I've learned so much from you all. Special thanks to Cyndi Lee for creating OM yoga, my first yoga home, and for her trust, confidence, and early support—without which none of this would have happened. Her words in the foreword have made this book complete.

I honor my OM yoga teachers Jennifer Brilliant and Dana Strong, who gave me solid yogic principles and taught me to "sit well"; all my colleagues, fellow yoga teachers, and studio staff of OM yoga; and yoga teachers both inside and outside the cancer community.

I give sincere gratitude to the dedicated y4c teachers who have helped keep the y4c weekly classes going over the past ten years and without which I could not take a vacation.

I'm thankful for the generosity of founders Stephanie Tang of Sacred Sounds Studio and Elena Brower of Virayoga and their respective staffs who provided the y4c program the comfort of space.

A huge thanks to Katie McKay for her talent and patience as my illustrator.

I thank my oncologists, Dr. Julie Olin and the late Dr. Jeanne Petreck, for their good work in keeping me alive.

Special thanks to Dr. Robyn Frankel-Tiger. The words of her foreword give depth to the purpose this book will have in the lives of future cancer patients and survivors.

One day I said to myself, "There is a book you need to write." Little did I know that it would take a village to complete it. My editorial support was extensive, spread over time and distance. I thank the good work of Ani Weinstein, Erin Teufel, Lara Rosenberg, and Neil Gordon for helping me launch this book. I was fortunate to have the gentle and competent editorial support of Meghan MacLean and Jeanie Levitan, from Inner Traditions & Bear and Company, to help get it to print.

All along the way, I had the constant and loving support of Jackson Kytle, who taught me the difference between a footnote and endnote. He was my captain of sentence smoothing, director of research, and is my life partner. There could never be too many words to thank Josi Kytle, my business partner and daughter. She marshaled her experience, talents, and strong stewardship to navigate the publishing world. She was selfless with her time and energy, protected me from just about everything she could, and gave me the confidence to make our ideas real. Both of their voices were a steady reminder that this book was important.

I am so grateful for the quiet support of my dear friends—Karen Armstrong; Susan Bloom; Paul Clausing; Jennifer Price; William Masciarelli; Sue Considine; Andi Pepper; Tara O'Reilly; Suzy Stevens; Lindsey Pearson; Mio Fredland; Edward Jones; my sister, Bernadette Prinster; my son, Ethan Kytle; and my daughter-in-law, Blain Roberts—all who would simply ask, "How's the book coming?"

Finally, thank you to those who have already gone and left part of their lives with me.

*"Just as the
caterpillar thought
her world had
come to an end, she
changed into
a butterfly."*

ANONYMOUS

Jean, cancer survivor

A Wellness Plan for Survival

I am a cancer survivor and certified yoga teacher, and the book you are holding in your hands will share what I have learned over more than a decade about cancer and yoga. *Yoga for Cancer* demonstrates why and how to use yoga to cope with cancer and cancer treatments. It describes a unique yoga methodology created to help cancer patients of all ages lessen treatment side effects—and enrich their lives. In the pages ahead, you will find inspiring stories, medical facts, and many practical exercises to help you regain and maintain your health.

Being diagnosed with cancer is like falling off your swing as a kid, face down into the mud, losing your breath, causing all the other kids to stop and stare in silence, and then having to walk home alone, covered in muck. You feel shocked, dirty, and most of all, alone. That is how I felt years ago when I found a lump and was diagnosed with stage 2 breast cancer. Today, all cleaned up and healthy for more than a decade, I lead a yoga program for cancer survivors.

Most people know that cancer treatments like chemotherapy can cause baldness and nausea. The treatments and their side effects can be as frightening as the disease itself, which is what my students say. Physical limitations, lifelong side effects, and vulnerabilities imposed by surgeries—all can be underestimated. Or perhaps we cannot really hear about side effects from our doctor when we are scared of dying.

When the treatments are finished, you go home, alone, to sort out the mess, with many more questions than answers. Doctors do not hand you a prescription for how to live the rest of your life. Western medical models are designed to cure disease and rarely, if ever, include a wellness plan for survival. *Yoga for Cancer* provides the concepts and yoga tools with which you can construct your own wellness plan.

Many challenges are discussed in the pages ahead and when I started out, I did not have the ideas I have written about. This book is a record of what I learned and wish I knew when it all began. Early in my own recovery journey, I began to see that yoga was helping my recovery in ways I did not fully understand at the time. Through my first yoga practice, I began to regain control of my life. I also grew spiritually in ways I never anticipated and, years later, I hope I've become a more compassionate person and a better human being. Eventually, yoga for cancer—what I call *y4c,* to refer to the specific methodology—became my calling because promoting yoga with cancer patients and yoga teachers is my daily passion, from dawn to dusk, most days of the week.

A crisis provokes change. A hidden positive in any life-threatening illness is the chance to make the crisis work for you, to use the threat to life as a gift to *transform* life. Yes, that sounds idealistic and, true, everyone wants to find his or her own path. You do not have to become a saint. But I have no doubt that using yoga to take control—taking your breath back from the disease—is the key to a high quality of life. We want to use the time we have as fully as possible. Yoga continues to be my personal survival tool.

Ten years ago I was frustrated by the lack of information about cancer and yoga. I looked everywhere but found little. I began to research and play with insights that led to new yoga teaching principles and discoveries about fundamental anatomical facts. At every stage of my research, students and teaching colleagues helped refine these ideas, and I am grateful for their support and many contributions. I have applied these guiding principles to classic yoga poses, focusing on the biological and psychological benefits to cancer survivors. What I have written is, I hope, an innovative methodology for using the ancient and rich resources of yoga to help you, the survivor, to reduce pain, get back to normal quickly, and feel good about yourself. Actually, I hope you will use the yoga tools I describe to create a "new normal," maybe even a *better* one with knowledge, awareness, hope, and joy.

So, yoga is my prescription for health and well-being. I make no claim that it is a cure for cancer, which is a complex biological disease with many, many variations. In my experience, the right approach to yoga provides powerful benefits that are described later. As I will discuss, cancer has large elements of chance to it, beginning with the devolution of single cells and the immune system's attempt to find and kill these deviant cells. As you know, some parts of cancer are difficult to control. But you can control how you respond to the diagnosis, how you feel about your body, and what you can do to try to heal it.

Yoga can teach you to strengthen the immune system as well as soften the worst effects of illness and treatments. As this book will explain, yoga can cleanse the body of toxins and regulate normal body functions by stimulating internal systems, such as digestion, posture, cardiovascular functions, lymphatic flow, and breathing. Yoga also helps us stabilize and relax the body while enhancing concentration, memory, balance, mental acuity, and tranquility. Is there any medication that can promise all that? Who would not take such a pill, with or without cancer? That is why I think of yoga as a prescription for reclaiming life and as a wellness plan for moving on to long-term health.

The chapters ahead will discuss common side effects of cancer treatments and how to adapt yoga to new physical limitations, whether short- or long-term. This book will help you find the right class and teacher, become aware of exaggerated claims made about yoga, and avoid risky yoga styles and poses.

Three phases mark everyone's cancer journey, starting with the first, *diagnosis*. When you first hear the word *cancer* from your doctor, it feels like time stops, even though it is only a second or two. Time just stops! *Navigating through treatments* is the second phase and here you have choices to consider, but with much less information than many of us want. Again, time seems to stretch out like taffy. The length of the recovery phase will vary with the treatment effects, preexisting physical conditions, and lifestyle. Frustrating as it is, no one can predict how long recovery will take or how you will feel. *Survivorship* is the third phase, which lasts a long time, we hope. To be precise, it lasts the rest of your life. Personally, I do not like the word *survivor,* but after diagnosis, that is what you are as long as you live. For each phase I will tell you about many suitable yoga practices that add quality to life. I hope you will use this book to tailor yoga to your personal needs and stage of recovery.

HOW THE BOOK IS ORGANIZED

This book has one goal: to pass on as much information about yoga and cancer as I have found. Chapter 1 begins with my story, showing how getting diagnosed with breast cancer, having surgery, and receiving Western forms of treatment triggered my curiosity about how to rebuild my life. Like every survivor, suddenly I had to confront deep, frightening questions about what cancer is, how it will change my life, what I can do to avoid a recurrence, and how I can fill my future with health and hope.

We all want to understand how cancer came into our lives. We ask why, and then seek useful information about its cause and prevention as we move forward to recovery. Chapter 2 looks into the nature and basic facts of cancer with a special focus on yoga. In a way, everyone lives with cancer or cancerous cells on a daily basis especially the older we get. As I will explain, this tenant is fundamental to understand the complexity of the immune system and how yoga can provide the necessary tools and support to prevent what we all know as "cancer."

Chapter 3 starts with the story of Sarah, who came to my yoga class hating her body, afraid to move, and skeptical. Slowly, she found the yoga tools she needed to create a wellness plan, one that changed her body image, fears about using her body, and doubts about yoga. Unlike other experiences in life, cancer makes us aware of our bodies. Unfortunately, this awareness means becoming attuned to every little pain or irregularity that before cancer we didn't notice or think much about. Treatments frighten us; surgery hurts. In the case of breast cancer, physical therapy after surgery is critical, and the survivor's insurance often only covers two weeks.

Few survivors get acquainted with a new version of their body in such a short time. We might ignore how surgery has compromised mobility, strength, and general ability to function over the course of many months, much less a lifetime. When treatments are over, oncology nurses, doctors, and insurance agents wish you well and turn to the next patient. The message becomes clear: It is up to you to prescribe the next steps on your journey! You need a wellness plan.

Chapter 3 shows you how informed, intelligent yoga offers a valuable set of tools for your wellness plan. I will provide you with some research and facts that explain key benefits of yoga such as building strength and mobility, detoxification, weight management, improved sleep, and many others. Ten benefits of yoga are described in detail. Understanding the *why* is the first step to making yoga part of any survivor's wellness plan.

The next section of the book—part 2—takes all the research and theory and puts it into action. It will provide you with the formula for making yoga a part of your normal routine and explain how to put these tools together as a practice. A *practice* is a set of actions routinely done daily, or almost daily, with the goal of self-improvement and growth. It's a word that has special meaning in the yoga world. Unlike a doctor who practices medicine, or a baseball player who practices with her team, a yoga practice is more like hygiene for the body and the mind. Just like you would not think of starting your day without brushing your teeth, a yogini would not end her day without finding a time and place for her personal yoga practice.

I will outline a formula to construct a yoga practice using ten basic elements or modules. The yogic goal of each module is different, and each is part of the overall goal of balancing all the body's systems. Together they create a complete practice based on your needs. Although precise and sequential, the elements are flexible and modular, taking into account the individual person, cancer, and other special conditions that we all have precancer. Each module is illustrated with examples.

Chapter 4 presents the y4c theory and chapter 5 describes how to begin a practice, focusing on practical issues such as creating the right time and space to conduct your home practice if you are not attending a yoga class. This section also introduces my recommendation for the basic building blocks from which your practice will be gradually developed, including key elements such as breathing and meditation. I also want you to understand how to vary your practice in order to motivate yourself and respect how your body is feeling on a given day.

Chapter 6 is the heart of the book because it is packed with illustrations of fifty-three yoga poses along with practical instructions for each pose or sequence. Survivors will want to tailor their practice to their physical needs, and this chapter tells you the poses to avoid or use only with caution. When you arrive at this chapter you will have all the elements with which to develop your own yoga practice.

Students who are new to yoga, especially those I meet on yoga retreats, ask for a guide to continue yoga on their own. Chapter 7 includes practice sequences for different levels and time lengths. The goal is to help you build your practice if you cannot find the right yoga class or there isn't a studio close by. All yogins* learn to build their practice around the practical constraints in daily life, which means you seldom have the perfect class, time, or place to practice. We do the best we can if only for five minutes a day or while walking to the subway or riding in the car.

Chapter 8 offers poses that address common physical and emotional side effects that cancer patients and survivors face, including lymphedema, bone

---

*The word *yogin* is a gender-neutral term for one who practices yoga. The masculine form is *yogi* and the feminine from is *yogini*.

loss, weight gain, anxiety, and insomnia. These categorized poses can provide the necessary tools for survivors to lead their own recovery as and when needed. They are also valuable tools for yoga teachers. Most yoga teachers are trained to teach a diverse and general population, but lack the specific knowledge to teach cancer survivors with their unique needs, concerns, and fears.

Survivors need resources. Given the isolating aspects of surviving cancer and the roller coaster of emotions experienced, connecting with other people helps the survivor heal both emotionally and physically. While readers 2,000 miles from New York City won't be able to chat with other survivors after my class, they *will* be able to take advantage of the online resources, foundations, hospitals, clinics, and retreats described in the Resources for Survivors section on pages 283–85. This section also includes my comprehensive website, www.y4c.com.

Yoga has changed my life, and I want to help others rebuild their lives. No one path exists through cancer to recovery. No perfect method can be recommended for building a personal yoga practice, much less a whole new life. Please use the ideas you read about in my book in any way that is useful for you. You are in charge, and that is the most important idea I have to share.

*Namaste.**

---

*This Sanskrit greeting is often used by yogins but has no direct English translation. The one I like goes like this: The best in me salutes the best in you.

PART 1

Understanding Cancer and the Benefits of Yoga

Hope is not a plan.

Tari Prinster

Every chapter in my book carries forward a conversation among three voices: first, my personal experience as a patient, survivor, and teacher; second, all that I have learned from my students and other yoga teachers about teaching survivors; and third, scientific principles from physics, biology, and psychology that have to guide our choices. We will draw on the best insights from Eastern traditions like Buddhism and yoga, but also the best current thinking in Western science. This book's careful integration of many traditions of living well and healing sets it apart from other approaches.

Sometimes the narrative will be personal, and at other times, our focus will shift to yoga—its great traditions and powerful tools. Throughout I return to the concept that you, the survivor, need to control your own cancer and recovery journey. That path, like your life, will be unique because the changes ahead and new life challenges are impossible to predict. That is why I believe basic insights and new tools for learning are so important. As much as possible I invite you to be your own doctor on the treatment team rather than a passive patient waiting for something to happen.

Like any serious challenge in life, cancer leads many people to think in new ways and to make better choices, like improving their diet or getting more exercise. Cancer propels us toward better health!

*Cancer steals
your breath,
yoga gives it back.*

TARI PRINSTER

Tari, cancer survivor

1

My Story

When the sun drifted behind the foothills near my childhood home in western Colorado, shadows from the cottonwood trees cooled the galvanized pipes my father had used to construct a set of climbing bars attached to our garage. The date would have been 1954 or earlier. Entertainment in those days was simple, like spending school vacation days hiking with my brothers or after-school hours irrigating the peach orchard. TV had not reached us yet and the only media entertainment was an occasional movie (I remember being terrified by *Bambi*) or listening on the radio to Bobby Benson and the B Bar B Riders. I was a skinny, wiggly kid who liked to hang by her knees on the monkey bars.

Alone in the backyard I would play on the monkey bars on summer evenings when I was nine or ten. I fell often and the thump to the ground knocked the breath out of me. I remember the second of panic and fear, struggling to breathe, but fully conscious that my legs and arms could carry me to the kitchen door, speechless and gasping, so that I could bury my head in my mother's skirt. I remember too that she would say, "It's going to be okay . . . Just breathe deeply." That same feeling of having the wind knocked out of me occurred again at age fifty-three when I heard these words: "You have cancer—invasive ductal carcinoma." That took my breath away! In a flash, the idea came to me: my life is threatened! The threat was real and in my face.

Those three little words—*invasive ductal carcinoma*—were only the beginning of many breathless moments. The parade of treatment options, decisions, side effects, medications, expenses, insurance forms, phone calls, and empty hours waiting for test results—all floated past like debris on a sea of uncertainty and anxiety. Perhaps you have already had this experience. No matter what kind or at what stage, cancer steals the breath, clouds the brain, and weakens the body. That same thump of hitting the ground, having lost my grip on the monkey bars while enjoying life as a kid, started me thinking I could never breathe again. Something was stuck, not working, and very wrong. Life could stop.

The word *cancer* pried loose my hold on life, and time just seemed to stop. At least it stopped until I took the next breath as a cancer survivor. Since then nothing has been the same.

Today, I wear a T-shirt with the words *Breathe Deeply: Appreciate the Moment.* But fifty years ago my mother had no idea her words would become part of popular culture. She was not a yogini. Certainly, back in those days the idea of yoga was not a term associated with healing or health. Perhaps there was a vague association with philosophy or religion. She had no idea. Today, our twenty-first-century Western concept of yoga is that it's a way to get a good stretch and acquire flexibility, or it's a meditation technique to let go of stress. While these are benefits of yoga, more subtle and less understood is the yoga principle of learning how to breathe. Sounds simple, right? Structured and careful breathing is the harness that unites the body and mind—and has the potential to heal. We'll learn more about breathing and health shortly.

What I learned from my mom, ever so simple and powerful, has become my lifelong tool for survival. Her words are a guiding principle for me and this book. Perhaps I would not have made the connection of my mother's wisdom to the teachings of yoga had I not been diagnosed ten years ago with breast cancer. Finding my breath, taking *back* my breath, was the beginning of the rest of my life.

I have shared parts of my personal experience because learning you have cancer is an intensely personal moment, raising so many deep feelings and fears. Shock, embarrassment, and anxiety can overwhelm. Relating parts of my experience, good and bad, may help my readers understand the path ahead, although everyone's journey will be unique, and every path will have smooth passages, sharp bumps, and sudden detours.

HARNESSING A HEALING BREATH

When I found out that I had serious breast cancer, I got angry. Cancer is a bag of surprises! The word *cancer* conjours up threatening images, like seeing the eyes of a hungry tiger as you open the door. We have not lost the biological connection to our ancestors who felt there are only two choices: run or get eaten! But where do you run in a New York apartment?

I have read how the hormone adrenaline, released at moments of shock, injury, or trauma, has an anesthetizing effect on the nervous system. This protective reaction allows us to do extraordinary things. It gives us the ability to not feel pain in the split second after an accident, to get up and walk away. Or it protects you from feeling fear when you risk your life to pull a child from the path of a speeding car.

Cancer is a cold new reality. No matter the type or stage of your cancer, you will survive the initial shock only to find yourself enrolled in Cancer Boot Camp. Medical terms, weird theories, and frightening statistics everywhere. No time to sort out personal emotions when you are dealing with life-and-death decisions.

 Let everything happen to you: beauty and terror.
Just keep going. No feeling is final.
RAINER MARIA RILKE

When you do find some time you may find yourself flooded with unaccountable, sometimes uncontrollable, emotions like anxiety or depression. Where did *that* come from, you wonder? Still, the emotions are not all negative. Quiet, reflective moments may surprise you when, if you listen carefully, the protective numbing gives way to contemplative, peaceful feelings. For me, however, the strongest emotion was anger. Why me? Why now? I don't have time for this. . . .

What made me mad was the timing. My kids were nearly out of the house and my professional life was taking off. I was not ready to stop, much less to think about the end game, or dying. Then, for an entire year, I fell into that dehumanizing process of being a "patient." I found myself treated differently by family and friends, who looked at me like I was sick even before my hair fell out. I just wanted to get back to "normal" as quickly as possible and not to have to stop and think about the meaning of life. I was living life and enjoying the progress I had earned among the challenges normally encountered as a woman of fifty-three. Not this, not now, why me? I was mad.

Anger is not unique to my situation. I hear my students get angry with their bodies or blame their willpower, as if to say, "My body betrayed me in spite of my being so good to it all these years." But I was not angry at my body. Yes, I had done all the right things: eaten all the veggies, jogged those miles, kept my weight below average, avoided dark feelings with a positive attitude, never took hormone replacement therapy . . . on and on. I had been a good girl. Thinking about the body this way, as something separate from us, perhaps like a bad friend who let us down, is understandable but not helpful. Rather, we need to think about cancer, treatment, and recovery in new ways, powerful ways that build resilience and improve quality of life.

A cancer diagnosis gives rise to strong emotions, for sure. Feelings of anger, guilt, and betrayal come without invitation. Put aside these emotions momentarily to focus on the cancer. Whether it is the inconvenience, as in my case, or the lack of discipline that makes you angry, we all want to find answers to the questions: What went wrong? Why do I have cancer? And we are soon frustrated to learn that there are still few answers to what really causes cancer, and how to cure it. You try to avoid it and, even though you follow health guidelines, you get it. Can it be that cancer is just random, a matter of chance? Yes, much of the time, is the sobering answer. Chapter 2 will cover the basics of cancer as a disease.

Cancer is sneaky. In so many ways, you feel defenseless. Not only do you lose your breath, you lose control: control of how you look and feel, how others respond to you, what your plans for the future will be, and even what you wear to the hospital. The way back from feeling powerless is to take charge in any way you can, as the following examples show.

Surgeries came first for me, three in total. The initial lumpectomy was not successful because a small-town surgeon hadn't gotten "clear margins," meaning that cancer cells could have been left behind, so that meant another surgery. I got mad again when I could not lift my arm after the sentinel node biopsy, another procedure I had in order to check if any cells had ended up in the nearest lymph node that then could spread to other parts of the body.

Cancer treatments make you think about the smallest details of daily life. I had worn a long-sleeved T-shirt to the hospital for that prodedure, but had to use a surgical scissor to cut it open because I could not raise my arm over my head to get it on. No one told me to wear a button-up front shirt! My reaction sounds like—and is—a small thing, but it conveys my feelings. I was mad that no one told me how to dress for cancer surgery.

One thing I was told that could happen after this particular procedure was the possibility of lymphedema, an uncomfortable, disfiguring, and physically limiting condition in which lymph fluid builds up in tissues, causing swelling. Some women respond to this possibility with fear stronger than that of dying, which suggests the strong emotions being felt. Once again I got mad and even more determined. I thought, no way was I going to develop lymphedema or live my life without my sport activities. To get my life back I needed to strike a bargain with my treatments.

So, two weeks after my last surgery and with my doctor's okay, I started back to yoga. Slow and gentle, of course, but with a different focus. What interested me was not what I could *not* do, but what I *could* do. Attention to other parts of my body that were healthy surprised me, like my legs, which seemed eager, ready to move and stretch. Of course, I wanted to get back to normal, but I began to notice a subtle shift in my thinking.

Activity was good for me and important in small doses, even at first. Soon I noticed how doing something as simple as lying on my back with my eyes closed and listening to soft music could change my mood (in yoga we call it *active resting*). Along the way I discovered things that I would have missed before getting cancer.

I learned to appreciate the ability to breathe. Now it felt so good to follow the movement of air through my throat and out my nose. I could not take a really deep breath that would expand the ribs, stretching the incisions around the surgical staples. But I was breathing mindfully, enjoying it—and I was doing my yoga. The idea of *active, intentional rest* was new to me, an opportunity to stop trying to be so athletic and to appreciate simple relaxation.

> *It has been said that life has treated me harshly; and sometimes I have complained in my heart because many pleasures of human experience have been withheld from me . . . if much has been denied me, much, very much, has been given me . . .*
>
> HELEN KELLER

Another idea slowly formed. I found myself motivated to detoxify my body of all chemicals that I had put into my body, so I could better tolerate chemo drugs. I used the time before starting chemotherapy like preparation for a marathon. Yes, I was scared, but I was going to be ready to fight. Partly, this is my personality, but this fight approach to cancer is also common. Perhaps it is easier for us to think of cancer as the enemy on a battlefield rather than feel powerless as a passive patient waiting to be cured. Imagining myself a warrior, I was masking my fears and all the uncertainty because I was not ready to show my family and friends all that I was feeling. Mask or not, the image of becoming a warrior gave me hope.

Rewards are a great motivation to get us through difficult tasks. Often I hear how my students use a reward strategy when going through cancer treatments: a special vacation to the beach, a cup of chocolate ice cream, perhaps tickets to a ball game with a grandchild. Before each chemotherapy treatment, I gave myself a gift of a yoga session with Tara, my yoga teacher and friend. Then I took my bottle of homemade ginger water, a sweater, and thick socks (the chemotherapy lounge was so cold!), and was off to my chemotherapy session.

It was simple to control what I did to comfort the body. But my mind was not so easily calmed. For example, my insight into the great potential of using mindful breathing started happening on my way to that first chemotherapy treatment. I began to experience my feelings of anger turn toward anxiety and vulnerability.

Fear of the unknown was another loss of control. I was so afraid of surrendering my body to the effects of the drugs even though, at the same time, I was just as convinced they would give me life. When my nurse began that first drip into my left arm, my heart began to pound, partly in response to the preload of antihistamines before the chemo is infused. Acute anxiety was a totally new feeling for me, another breathless moment.

Fear is not pleasant, and feeling vulnerable is hard for me. Anxiety causes muscles to tighten, palms to sweat, and your mouth gets dry as blood pressure and respiration rates elevate. I could feel this happening. My heart rate was out of control! Was I breathing? No! Gone again, that critical supply of life-giving oxygen, just by thinking about something like chemotherapy that is designed to save lives.

I needed to take charge. Anxious or not about chemo, I was not going to withdraw from treatment, but all the emotional side effects were not part of the deal. Finding a way to manage them was going to have to come from deep inside. Looking back, like so many others I had found the will to fight when challenged. I learned that human beings are resilient and this resilience was pivotal to my recovery.

I can still hear my mother say, when I ran into the house excited to tattle on one of my brothers' misdeeds, "Take a breath and start over," or "Count to ten and tell me again." I counted my steps to the chemo easy chair in that freezing room. I counted my breaths between each drip. The mind follows the breath. It is so simple. A relaxed mood and calm mind cannot be maintained if you are gasping for breath. Likewise, an agitated, irritable mood will be soothed by a long, smooth breathing pattern. Nothing can be more deeply comforting than the willful, conscious movement of air in and out of soft, expandable lung tissue. In chapter 2 I will describe exactly how the mechanics of breathing affect the nervous system, and readers can use the new knowledge to regain control of their feelings. This insight about the breath became the first principle of my blend of yoga for cancer—the y4c methodology. Cancer may have taken away my breath, but I took it back. And so can you.

HOW I FOUND YOGA

People ask me how I got into yoga. I like to say it was for the "wrong reason"—vanity! It was shortly after my fiftieth birthday, that half-century milestone marker. Life is a sequence of milestones. Think about it. What is a milestone? To measure intervals between important places, the Romans used stone markers along their many roads and viaducts across continents they conquered. Milestones provide the traveler with a reference, indicating the remaining distance to a destination. For the most part, this should be reassuring and a guide that you are preceding nicely and in the direction desired. Milestones along our life journey carry us forward with anticipation; once passed, they can become joyful memories—or opportunities, at least—to learn something new.

Different milestones appear on our chosen paths according to particular ambitions or needs. But all of us share the certain ones like first birthday and first step, and for women: first menstrual period and first hot flash. Like most women, the milestone of menopause for me was important. "It's all downhill from here!" seemed to be the only attitude I garnered from my mother, friends who had been through it, or those images in popular culture. My first hot flash happened in 1995.

Before that I saw little escape from the wrinkles, saggy skin, thinning hair, and blurry restaurant menus. In our twenty-first-century Western world, all these inevitable challenges of aging can be eased by cosmetic surgery, a pill, or a pair of designer glasses. A huge decision for me was whether to use hormone replacement therapy (HRT). The allure of this pill or patch was that all my youth could be returned. Most of my friends were taking some form of HRT. Even my mother did twenty-five years earlier and my younger sister had been on HRT for ten years.

Nineteen years ago I was not sure. My skepticism was intuitive, not supported by research in 1995. HRT was just not for me! I had two kids in the 70s big wave of natural childbirth. That seemed right then, so why not go through menopause drug free as well? Taking an artificial hormone so my periods would continue for an undetermined length of time when I was way past my childbearing years, all in order to avoid night sweats, seemed senseless. Back then no one knew what hormone therapy was doing—or could do—to the body long-term because the treatment had not been around long enough. If research existed, I didn't know about it. Women felt better using them.

So why not? To me, it seemed that everything about HRT in 1995 was inconclusive. There were other postmenopausal conditions: weight gain, heart disease, bone loss. Research suggested that these conditions were manageable, even preventable with diet and exercise. Besides, menopause is not a disease. It is a life milestone. So I made the choice to get through it without drugs. And I embraced yoga to help me manage the side effects and smooth the journey into my next chapter.

So in 1995, committed to the goal of managing my menopause symptoms without drugs, I was going regularly to the gym. On the milestone of my fiftieth birthday I was on my way to the gym when I noticed my reflection in the window of a car. In the reflection I saw my grandmother's hunched shoulders and my mother's curving spine. True, I was already seeing wrinkles, but in that moment I saw the silhouette of an old woman, me! That was when I realized I needed to do something more than jog and lift weights. Passing through the reproductive years, the hormonal shifts were happening, no fault of mine. Correcting the curve of my spine was *my* job. Few things provide more motivation than vanity.

Soon I began to notice that even young people who slumped looked old; but, at no matter what age, people who did yoga had good posture. Getting old was as much about *looking* old as *feeling* old. As a complement to my other activities, I started practicing yoga at age fifty in the Bikram and ashtanga yoga traditions to get what seemed like the best benefits as fast as possible. Even at twice a week, I could see my body change in ways that other conditioning exercises had failed. My posture improved and I began to lose the belly fat fold. My stamina, mental focus, and coordination—all were getting stronger.

I thought it was due to being postmenopausal, but my moods fluctuated less. And my bowels were regular, an often unspoken benefit of yoga. My curiosity about all these benefits at the time was minimal, maybe because my motive was simple vanity. Only when cancer came into my life did I begin to ask the deeper questions of why my body was responding to this form of exercise more quickly and favorably than it had in the past to traditional exercise and sports. In my mind, cancer raised these questions of *how* and *why*.

During chemotherapy treatments I was amazed at the number of times I was told by family and friends to "take it easy." However well-intended, this advice fed my new identity as "cancer patient," and made me feel like an invalid. I didn't like this image nor find it helpful. My desire to feel normal was as strong as my vanity. The late writer and journalist Christopher Hitchens put it this way—"To be a cancer survivor means you lose your citizenship in the Land of the Well, and wake up as a foreigner in a new country called Cancer Land."* I wanted to continue my physical activities, and I did so to a reasonable

---

*The late Christopher Hitchens wrote about the "new land" of a cancer patient with its strange facts and difficult words in "Topic of Cancer," *Vanity Fair* (September 2010).

extent. The approach was to do something every day, even if I didn't feel like it, *especially* on chemo day.

I was on a weekly treatment schedule as part of a clinical trial I had joined that left me six other days of the week to fill with healing activities. Living in Vermont then, it was easy to walk or bike along a nearby recreation path. When the weather was bad my yoga mat was a fine place to stretch and create movement in my body fluids. That was the key! I became obsessed with the idea of moving the chemo drugs through and out of my body as quickly as possible. I had no clue as to whether exercise would do this. But it seemed like the right thing.

If you have been in chemotherapy, you know the feeling of drowsiness when you walk out of the clinic or hospital after sitting in a chair for three to five hours. For me, moderate exercise was a welcome relief. For most of us, the feeling of chemo fatigue is cumulative and as I moved through nearly ten months of treatments, it became necessary to modify my walks, rides, and time on the yoga mat. Doing some kind of moving can take many forms, even if it is just sensing movement in a resting yoga pose as we will explore in chapter 3.

Here is how I did yoga during those months of chemo. My living room had several floor-to-ceiling windows that looked out onto a Vermont valley framed by tall trees, opening to a western sky. I gave my yoga mat a permanent place in front of those windows. That spot was my place and became the anchor of my daily routine, the sanctuary of self-healing. That healing space was always there, inviting me back to breathe, to move, and to quiet my mind.

My chemo treatments started during the green of summer, 2000. As the months passed so did the seasons, and from my window perch I could follow nature's cycles of life . . . green to golden reds and then, winter white. The pattern in that rise and fall seemed to hide a silent secret. Each day was different with chemo and cancer, just like every session on my yoga mat I modified to match my energy. I created a yoga routine that started usually in the evening after work by sitting comfortably on my mat.

Most of the week I was alone, so being quiet was possible. Closing my eyes, I would wait, looking for signs of life in my body, like my quiet stomach, tingling hairless head, or heaviness in my bones—anything that *felt*. Then I watched my thoughts buzz about my mind. I tried not to respond to any of these feelings or thoughts. This could last for several minutes, or a few seconds. I began to move in rhythm with my breath doing small, slow gestures. Eventually, small movements became large ones. I followed patterns I had learned in various yoga classes, but nothing identifiable as any particular yoga style. I did what felt right.

Some days the movements would take me into vigorous balances and energetic poses, weaving a choreography between them. Or I would spend sixty minutes doing this quasi-dance, or just rolling around from pose to pose with little pauses for as long as it was pleasant. Other days I would get comfortable and become so still I could hear my heartbeat.

What I am trying to say is that mindful movement is healing, and so is stillness and rest, if we let ourselves sink into the peace. For one thing, hearing a heart muscle move is enough proof that there is some kind of movement going on deep inside, because there is always movement in the body even when we are not moving. Movement is a sign of life. CPR training uses simple diagnostics that check for movement. Is the chest rising and falling with the movement of air through the lungs? Can you hear a heartbeat? Movement is *critical* to good health and the cornerstone of my second principle, discussed in chapter 4 on pages 84–85.

When I finish my mat time I always enjoy a long pause. This is the ceremonial last pose of Savasana—final resting position. During seven months of chemo my daily practice varied in frequency, duration, and intensity as the challenges of my recovery unfolded.

MOVE TO LIVE, LIVE TO MOVE

My simple yoga practice helped me in ways I could not anticipate and became my personal tool for survival. It started with a simple idea, "I need to move every day on my way through treatments and to recovery." I stopped using the gym treadmill, but I did not stop moving. As you read further we will explore how and why movement in yoga aids recovery.

Movement of any kind means we are alive! Finding the right kind of movement for your personal situation is the challenge. With or without cancer, our bodies are made to move. Quality of life and healthy longevity depend upon daily movement.* Without exercise muscles and bones weaken rapidly, so it's important to "use it or lose it." Without exercise the body stagnates and gets dull and weak. The mind too! Moving keeps both fresh. I live to move and I move to live *better*.

What kind of exercise is best? I have to answer my own question. Yoga is better! But *how* and *why* is it better? I went looking for answers myself as my

---

*Both theory and clinical research by national associations like the American Cancer Society (ACS) support the physical and mental health benefits of even moderate exercise over the life span. Exercise can help with weight control, and being overweight is a risk factor for cancer. More is being learned about ideal exercise frequency as well as the exact biological mechanisms. Even a modest amount of exercise seems to help.

story continues. My body was changing from this cancer challenge, and so was my mind.

WHY WE ASK QUESTIONS

When the diagnosis conversation starts, doctors explain the basics: what is a tumor, why it should be removed, how that is done, and what happens after that. It all happens so fast and so much of the new vocabulary is foreign; that is why I took a tape recorder to early sessions with my surgeon and oncologist. The doctors sent the tumor and me to the lab. After all those tests I got a picture of all my internal body parts, not just my breasts, but my lungs, kidneys, ovaries, bowels, and even my pancreas. Cancer Boot Camp, Basics 101! I had no idea how many lymph nodes lived in my body, or where they were. Seeing my entire lymphatic system lit up with a radioactive isotope was an opportunity to see myself differently. I was able to look *inside* the body—*my* body—and see it in a new way.

So when chemotherapy started I found myself in a crash course on immunology, or how cell biology works. Frankly, I had never thought about the balance of my white and red blood cells before, or how they quietly work making blood and its several protective agents that are all the time guarding me from infections and disease—keeping me alive.

All this new learning only sharpened my questions as I watched my hair fall out, and asked why, again. Nurses were willing to explain things like special care for post-surgery drains. Technicians showed me how the direction of the radiation beam would bypass my heart and lungs (or so they hoped). I saw the inside of my body through X-rays, blood tests, and sonograms. And I was getting some of the science behind cancer.

Cancer became the teacher of a motivated learner! I began to look inside this wonderful container—my body—and to see it from the inside out. If the body is a car, I had never bothered to look under the hood, or to ask how it worked or what made it break down. I had not gone looking for an owner's manual, but was finding one all the same.

Something else was happening as another question arose: If I was learning all this about my body, what was going on in my mind? What I saw inside my body beneath the skin was not as scary as I had imagined. However, thinking about the potential of cancer cells growing elsewhere in my body was unsettling, for sure. I was beginning to grasp the impermanence of life. Death was no longer simply an idea or abstraction, and thoughts about it became an unavoidable part of daily life.

I was in Cancer Boot Camp training to be a *warrior*, odd as that term might seem to people outside the cancer community. I didn't ask to attend, of course, and the experience is not something I would choose again or recommend. But adversity can be used for good. I was being prepared for the rest of my life, and it was then that I began to realize that the choices I made about how I treated my body *today* would improve quality of living *tomorrow*.

Going through chemo made me tired. I expected that, but didn't anticipate the cumulative effect and, toward the end, how bone-weary I would feel. At the same time I seemed to grow emotionally stronger. Science measures the side effects of cancer drugs by the symptoms they produce and the length of time those drugs prolong a life. Could that same science measure the emotional strength of a survivor after treatments? As cancer was making me a warrior, something else was happening to me. Another kind of wisdom was unfolding. At the time I was not sure what to call it. But its presence was felt deep inside— in my body and in my mind.

Even as I gathered strength and energy after completing chemotherapy, my desire to return to what had been normal physical activities like the bike and the gym waivered. I felt something very different in my body. What was this difference? I wanted to do more yoga because when I left my mat, not only did my body feel good, so did my mind.

Cancer was teaching my body and mind how to work together more closely. I had not been listening before, or paying attention to my vital signs in the way that cancer was teaching me now. A new kind of body-mind wisdom had developed during those months of treatments—to feel, sense, question, and know my body in such different ways. All this learning through cancer was happening. My yoga practice was leading me to profound insights, slowly and quietly, about my body and mind—especially the complex way in which they interact.

When my two weeks of insurance coverage for physical therapy ended, things I did on my yoga mat were more helpful than therapy in increasing my range of motion. It is said that nerve sensation in the arm after axillary node surgery is not likely to return. But the feeling in my right armpit was returning. On a more discreet level, the discomfort of constipation—chemo's best-kept secret—was eased with yoga.

The great comfort of meditation became clear to me as a concrete, practical therapy, something I had not entirely appreciated prior to cancer. I needed it and I was feeling its potential as a self-healing tool. There was great value in being able to quiet my thoughts when trying to go to sleep at night, or coping with the stress of waiting in the doctor's office for the results of my follow-up exams, or lying alone with my fears inside an MRI machine for forty-five minutes. I could feel the direct effects on my nervous system.

Meditation combined with breathing was a powerful relaxation technique, just as the yoga masters suggested. I needed to know how all this was working in *my* body. The hidden, positive side of a life-threatening disease like cancer is that it gets our attention and if we respond with purpose, it can lead our minds and bodies to a better quality of life.

WANTING TO UNDERSTAND

Was this a miracle, or was there a science to yoga? Early on, I was skeptical about the claims made about yoga, choosing to ignore the "yoga-speak" about its "healing powers." Now, yoga was doing that for me . . . I could feel it! I was experiencing change in my body and in my emotional resilience. I wanted to know more, and I set out to explore the yoga community and to experiment.

That is when I started reading about the biological effects of yoga on the body, asking how and why yoga could affect cancer and promote recovery. I was not willing to just accept that yoga worked. I studied the lymphatic system, learning how deep belly breathing can directly affect the system's efficiency in detoxifying the body. At first I questioned the claim about detoxifying body twists—only to learn the fundamental physics of fluids and gravity that are involved! I was reading about the medical foundations of cancer, merging what I was learning into my growing knowledge of the science behind yoga.

When I was trying to learn everything I could about cancer, about yoga, and about cancer and yoga together, I went to many different types of yoga classes and read every book or article I could find. Less than a year into my recovery in 2001 I had the good fortune to live in New York City to continue my quest for the link between cancer and yoga. Here I used the city as my laboratory, studying anatomy and sampling every yoga style and any class offered for cancer survivors.

Expecting to find answers, I found myself disappointed by the cursory reference to cancer, the lack of understanding about the effects of cancer treatments on the body and, worse, a casual attitude about potential risks of injury. The yoga world seemed less based on science, more on generalities and hope. Some claims sounded unlikely, such as how a backbend could tone my abdominal organs, or a twist would detoxify my kidneys. In addition, if I had lost thirty lymph nodes, how would yoga strengthen my immune system? I wanted to know what yoga poses would ease the discomfort caused by lost body parts from cancer surgeries.

Clear answers regarding cancer were not coming from teachers, classes, or books written from a Western perspective about why things worked. Using my body, my mat, and lots of curiosity, I began to weave connections between biological facts, scientific studies, and the needs of cancer survivors into a collection of specific yoga poses designed to aid recovery.

As I got stronger I found some answers. My understanding of the connections between yoga and cancer grew. It became obvious that sharing this body of knowledge and wisdom with other survivors was the next step.

I decided to enroll in a yoga teacher training. That was 2002. Today, I lead a yoga for cancer program. It started with a simple idea: Yoga works! A kind of ministry began for me, one that today includes yoga classes targeting all cancers in all stages, retreats focused on learning how to use yoga as a tool to get back to normal, and accredited training workshops for certified yoga teachers. All this is based on a set of yoga teaching principles I have created that apply fundamental anatomical facts to classic yoga poses. This emerged from my search for answers as I felt my own body heal and change. It was what I prescribed for myself and what I offer to you in this book. This methodology is the cornerstone of y4c teacher trainings.

IT'S EASIER WHEN YOU ARE NOT ALONE

Doing it alone limits recovery. There is strength in community. Much of my type A personality has been revealed so far in my story. Certainly I have felt, and still feel, the cultural pressure to always be doing something. Some label this as mindless, not mindful, activity—going through life staying busy, as if that makes one feel more alive. Was I keeping busy so I did not have to think about cancer? Like so many of my students, I acted as if cancer was only happening to me. And I could work my way through all the struggles on my own terms, alone, as if there were no obstacles. But I did run into walls. At these junctures I learned not only to take a breath, meditate, and be a warrior prepared to face anything, but also that I was not alone. I had family and friends. They were there for me, offering wonderful support.

I discovered something else. In Cancer Land you need to connect to other people with cancer. Survivors speak a different language and connect on a different level.

The summer of 2000 I felt stigmatized with my bald head from chemo that I only covered with a baseball cap, just like my friend Alex (a wig is too hot, especially in summer). Alex was the younger brother of my daughter's high school friend and we became unlikely companions. At a very young age he had had a kidney transplant requiring almost fifteen years of immunosuppressive drugs that eventually caused his blood-related cancer. We would sit on his porch drinking tea, watching the deer wander in and out to eat from his garden, sharing a common field of grace, in Sanskrit called *sangha*. Loosely translated, sangha means "truth company," or "being in the company of the wise." Buddhist texts consider it to be one of *the* great doorways to inner freedom. Two is enough to make a sangha. The more you practice in this field of grace, the more likely you are to experience its power. You don't need words or special activities—and you do not have to join an existing community. Some of the most powerful healing communities are the ones we create informally.

Research shows the value of support groups for cancer patients and survivors. This is not everyone's cup of tea, however. Many people come to my yoga class as referrals from talk therapy groups. A yoga class can function like a therapeutic community, but with less talk. Still, as social creatures, humans benefit from sociability. We humans need each other.

Community and sangha refer to life outside the self, in the world, and engaged with others. It is the connection that goes beyond my "container," out of my sheath, and living in the world outside of the intense self-focus that cancer can cultivate. The shock of a cancer diagnosis can send people into a sheltering cocoon of isolation. Feeling part of a group can gently break through the terrible loneliness. One student put it this way, "At first I was scared I wouldn't fit into this yoga class. But I found myself in a room full of sisterly love, courage, endurance, and recovery. In that room I knew I was safe." This is a tiny example of the fears and scars each of these women carried with them—through every door they walked through, not just into yoga class. It is so much easier to navigate Cancer Land when you are not alone. It is a way to treat cancer from the inside out.

YOGA AND CANCER

My story continues with the stories of all the women, my students, from whom I have learned that yoga works. Their patience has allowed me to observe the many benefits of yoga through their bodies and in their personal healing. They come with curiosity, hope, and a willingness to be partners in a joint exploration. They come with fear, doubts, and questions about both cancer and yoga. It gives me great joy to have some answers, to witness how yoga helps them, and to be part of this cancer community that is full of sharing, support, and hope.

The questions and fears my students bring to class are important, an indication of being ready to move beyond the isolation of one's personal cancer. Cancer *is* scary. So is chemotherapy or surgery. Even yoga can be frightening to some people. All the mysteries of life are unsettling unless we learn to appreciate new learning. We can take some of that mystery away with knowledge and wisdom, through breathing, movement, and community.

One of my students, Tina, had been recently diagnosed with breast cancer and she was afraid to come to class before her mastectomy. She had heard that exercise and moving would spread her cancer (not true). My students share many secrets with me and with each other, one of the most common being that weight-bearing poses can cause lymphedema. Even though research shows otherwise, this misconception continues to create unnecessary worry about doing yoga.

MY NEW LIFE AS A YOGA TEACHER

Teaching a yoga class can be a mystery and frightening too. It is a race with the clock and a roller coaster for the mind and body. The seventy-five minute class for women cancer survivors is every Tuesday at 3:45 p.m. in a room called Sun. For me, class actually starts at 3:15, when I take the elevator up to the studio. By 3:20 many women survivors are waiting patiently.

I joyfully greet Tina, whom I have not seen in the past eight months due to work conflicts, new metastasis, and lymphedema in her right arm. Obviously, we needed to catch up. She looks happy, has better color, and is wearing the lymphedema sleeve that many women dread. In all of fifteen seconds I learn about her new treatment and new side effects. Behind her brave smile I sense great fear and suffering.

At 3:32 I hug Denise. Her bald head is not covered by the usual wig. I sense something is different—no, something is wrong! Ninety seconds later I know about her chemo setbacks, new drug protocol, her husband's affair and departure, and her father's hospitalization. That sadness is compounded by the fact that she is unable to visit her father because her immune system is too compromised with the new chemo. She begins to cry and I hug her again, assuring her that leaving class early to make a scheduled radiation appointment is okay. Denise has brain cancer.

By 3:35 the number of new faces has grown to four. The yoga studio is full of chatter, giggles, greetings, questions, stories, advice, and sisterly love. The students are like kids in the playground during recess, not women facing a life-threatening disease, long-term disfigurement, and disability. Friends settle mats next to friends they only see in my class. They make room for each other, eagerly advising new students how to set up, what to expect. The room is full of energy. Are these cancer survivors, or a group of preteens getting ready for a sleepover, I ask myself. Today there are twenty-four warrior women lying on mats in ninety-degree heat: eight are undergoing chemo treatments; three are recovering from surgeries within the last three months; two have serious lymphedema; one is taking medication for seizures; and half have some form of breast reconstruction.

Time to teach yoga! I draw a blank. Every time, at the start of class, this happens. For more than ten years I have taught at least one weekly class for women cancer survivors and every time the first seconds fill me with anxiety. Why is this class so hard to teach?

As I fumble over my words to explain the first pose, the women immediately quiet, listen, and gently prepare in silence. I feel they afford me respect I do not deserve. My mind is still a blank. Eventually, everyone gets settled and calm, including me. In the stillness and quiet we collectively begin to do yoga by bringing awareness to the breath. Unrestricted breathing in and breathing out. Oh, so nice!

Some of the calmest moments in my life happen on a crowded, noisy subway. The sensory distraction forms an envelope, a sheath, around me. The overload becomes the invitation into a soft internal space where I feel at ease in the surroundings, just like now in the protection of our yoga cancer community. For several minutes I watch twenty-four reclining bodies breathe as smiles begin to appear on faces. The heavy baggage of individual cancer journeys falls away, a shared yoga journey begins.

With gentle warnings for those with recent surgeries, we begin to move mindfully and I introduce today's class theme: "Scars: the ones from cancer, the ones from life. How can we use both to be stronger?"

I lift my arm to show my scars and demonstrate the muscle groups affected by auxiliary node surgery. After I quickly explain where lymph nodes are located before removal and the directional flow of lymphatic fluids, we begin a series of anti-lymphedema, self-massage techniques. Pausing frequently to check for fatigue and offer adjustments to poses, I talk about the variation of sensation we now live with daily, the discomfort caused by resulting scar tissue, and why we need to stretch the pectoralis major muscle (anterior chest muscle)—specifically and constantly—to maintain or increase range of motion.

By now, I have used the C word several times. We cover the whole cancer vocabulary: scars, chemo, suffering, side effects, pain, and danger! While all these words may arouse fear for students in a normal yoga class, getting the word *cancer* into class acknowledges the silent elephant in the room, and doing so is therapeutic.

When I started looking into yoga classes for cancer survivors, I wondered why yoga teachers never said the word *cancer*. Instead, they use the words *relax* or *feel peaceful* frequently. Ironically, these pleasant words sent my mind racing into thinking about dying. To me, it was not healing to avoid the very reason the class was offered.

My students seem comforted by the exchange of questions we have when I first meet them as to what kind of cancer they have, how long they've had it, the treatments and side effects, and how it's going with their recovery. The relief students feel that their teacher is not afraid to acknowledge their illness creates a deep spiritual connection in the group that says, *We are all in this together.* When the class includes an explanation of how yoga breathing will assist in cleansing the immune system, and why that is important for reducing the risk of cancer recurrence, the response is a smile with each inhale. Talking about cancer can be uncomfortable, but not talking about it in frank terms makes cancer a terrifying mystery.

Finally, with fifteen minutes left, it all comes together. I return to the theme about scars. My eyes follow the shape of each reclined body. No struggling now. There are many smiles. I know all are in a safe, private place. Their scars, now hidden by T-shirts and baggy yoga pants, are body armor providing protection, a momentary escape from the challenges of their separate cancer paths. Like warriors, they have achieved the mighty throne from which to observe their bounty of self-care and healing. No battle is survived unscathed. These are the wounds that give life. No words needed.

The glow on each woman's face is the goal of yoga. Not some kind of nirvana, not profound enlightenment, not even heightened awareness. We find simple contentment in the bliss of *anandamaya kosha*, the most spiritual level of the body that yoga aids in healing, as discussed in chapter 4 on pages 87–88.

I hope the questions I have raised so far have captured your curiosity about how and why yoga works, the benefits of yoga, and how you can use yoga to reclaim your life during and after cancer. But before we race ahead, here are more questions. Throughout my story there are references, specific and subtle, to yoga principles that ground my thinking. What are they? How do they connect to my story and form the insights of y4c yoga?

Thousands of yoga poses and breathing techniques exist. All are important and, if used carefully, bring the benefits of yoga to a cancer patient and survivor. But how do we proceed in a mindful way to select, learn, and enjoy them? Like most learning tasks inherent in all bodies of knowledge, organizing principles are useful tools. We need some theory to guide our new learning. In chapter 2 we'll explore the scientific principles and published research that support yoga for those who have been touched by cancer and all who are living with cancer.

*Think with
the part of your mind
you call your body.*

ANI WEINSTEIN

yoga4cancer class in New York City

2

The Science of Cancer and Yoga

At some time in life every family will be visited by some type of cancer, partly due to the fact that people are living longer. According to the American Cancer Society, *lifetime risk* refers to the probability that a person will develop or die from cancer over a lifetime. In the United States, men have slightly less than a one in two risk; for women the risk is a little more than one in three.* In 2012 about 13.8 million Americans were living with cancer and/or cancer treatments' side effects, and as mortality rates continue to decline while incidence increases, in the next ten years the survivor population will grow by 24 percent.[1]

The chance of beating cancer or managing it better is improved if it's caught early—but like too many health problems, early detection can be less likely if one is poor, lives in a rural area, or is nonwhite.† Our culture's collective fear of cancer—not to mention the fear of dying for any reason—has led to information and misinformation being shared about

---

*For current information, see the American Cancer Society (ACS) website: www.cancer.org. For a general discussion, see also George Johnson, *The Cancer Chronicles* (New York: Alfred A. Knopf, 2013).

†An online BBC report cites research that young black women in the United Kingdom are more likely than their white counterparts to be diagnosed with advanced breast cancer with a poorer prognosis. See www.bbc.co.uk/news/health-24624517?print=true.

types of cancers that are out there, available forms of treatment, and, most significantly, the causes of cancer. The increasing spirit of openness about cancer is better than denial, not acknowledging it, or not being able even to say the word. It is a start, but we still have fears to manage and so much to learn about cancer and how to live well with it.

In this chapter we explore facts and science—answers to questions like: What is cancer really? How does it happen? and most importantly, How can yoga be a powerful tool on the path to recovery as well as an aid in prevention and avoiding recurrence? Let's look at the science that connects cancer and yoga.

A good prescription for an illness needs two things: an underlying science or organized way of thinking—whether it is Western, Eastern, or complementary medicine—and an educated doctor to write it. In this case, you become the doctor and the recommendation is yoga. As the doctor in charge, you want to give yourself a prescription that alleviates symptoms, reduces anxiety, strengthens your body, and most importantly, cultivates a new lifestyle to maximize the quality of your life and minimize the odds of cancer recurrence. This book is dedicated to helping you write one part of that prescription—yoga!

LIFE'S (LITTLE) MYSTERIES

Life is a mystery and so is cancer. Western science has tried to understand and explain these two mysteries—and progress is being made. Most of us know that a cancer starts with a chance mutation in one cell that then multiplies unchecked and competes with healthy normal cells for body resources. We understand that several hundred cancers exist with different properties and behaviors, and that treatment plans for the same cancer type vary vastly because a cancer evolves in each person in unique ways. We are learning that increasingly effective treatment can be individualized to a person's genetic profile. In spite of being a disease with a bad reputation, research continues.*

So where do *you* start? You just received the unthinkable: a cancer diagnosis. Being diagnosed with cancer sets you on the fast track for a doctorate from "Cancer University." So many questions, so little time, so much anxiety! You

---

*To read all the current research about cancer prevention and treatment and the many controversies is challenging for scientists, and even more so for laypeople. I recommend following the latest research from national and federal agencies like the National Cancer Institute (www.cancer.gov). Two recent books are worth reading for background: Clifton Leaf's *The Truth in Small Doses* about exaggerated claims made for improved treatment, and Siddhartha Mukherjee's acclaimed biography of cancer, *The Emperor of All Maladies*.

may ask, "Why me? What caused it? How do I get rid of it? How do I prevent its growth or recurrence?"

These are difficult questions, of course, but consider this: A cancer diagnosis opens doors for us! We can use the threat to motivate ourselves to learn how our bodies and minds work, and most importantly, to use the danger to question how we think about our diet, exercise, and level of stress along with life priorities in general. When we are frightened patients just learning about cancer, we may neglect to ask our doctors simple questions about cancer—what it is, how we got it, how we get rid of it!

Asking what causes cancer gives us information about the critical question of prevention and avoiding recurrence or developing new cancers. Most importantly, asking questions helps us think about how to experience life and the time we have left as fully as we can.

Often, the most important question—What is cancer?—is not asked. In Greek the word *cancer* means "crab," a creature with claw-shaped legs, moving in all directions. But cancer, of course, is not a crawly creature that somehow finds its way inside the body.

Here is a better metaphor: a cancer cell acts like an out-of-control teenager! It is hyperactive and grows really fast; it leaves stuff all over the house; and it breaks rules. In all these ways, cancer is sneaky, selfish, and stubborn.

Still you may think, "What is cancer?" What cancer is *not* can be the start of understanding what it is. That takes undoing the old thinking like we get cancer the same way we get a cold or headache, or that cancer is uncontrollable rather than being a manageable disease, which it is more and more. Both these mind-sets have wrong implications: that some foreign creature has entered the body from somewhere else, that it is not part of our body, and that the rest of the body will just stand by, watching it take over.

Let's start with thinking about cancer in new ways, like a scientist would— thinking about it as a puzzle and asking questions about how a particular cancer behaves. Okay, it is life threatening, but how does it act? How does it evolve in the body and how does it respond to our treatments to eliminate it or manage its growth? We want to think systematically.

I have learned that life and cancer share many things. Both are phenomena that science tries to explain and to control by looking at actions and complex processes, like how water that falls from clouds somehow makes its way into underground streams, into oceans, and then back up to the clouds to fall again. To understand how cancer behaves, surprisingly or not, we start by looking at how any living thing behaves—its patterns and complex interactions—especially at the cellular level.

Cancer, rather than being a disease coming from a common cause and having the same symptoms in every person, manifests itself uniquely in each person. This chapter will demonstrate the value of understanding the nature of your specific condition, and set you on the path to reclaiming your health and hope.

To understand cancer, we start with our own conception and growth as human beings. As we know, every human starts with the binding together of two cells: one egg cell (ovum) from mom and one sperm cell from dad. Call it a mystery or a miracle, from that moment on this unique coupling of cells begins to divide, each cell giving birth to another that contains the same unique genetic coding. Two cells grow to four, then eight, then sixteen, thirty-two, sixty-four, and so on until a complete body is formed. It is estimated that a fully grown adult human contains seventy-five to a hundred trillion cells! Dancing all together, each cell is programmed by its genes as far as what to do, how to divide, and how to become an eye or a toe. Eventually, this mass of dividing, differentiating cells becomes a complete human body composed of interlocking biological systems that have evolved for one purpose: to protect life!

At the moment of birth when the doctor slaps your bottom, you take your first breath. The diaphragm muscle begins to move and the rib cage expands and the lungs fill with air. All your interconnected body systems function seemingly without conscious effort. Blood flows, bringing oxygen to every cell, because your heart pumps it everywhere. The brain sends signals up and down the spine and to every extremity. Your stomach churns, hormones dash about. While all this occurs, a powerful immune system develops that we need to understand.

Cells do not last forever. From the moment of conception, the mom and pop cells give birth to the next generation. The "parental unit" has a job and a life span just like all parental units in life. They give birth to baby cells like themselves, maintain a good life, then die according to the laws of nature. Every cell is constantly being replaced. During that time, each cell has performed a function in the interest of creating a whole being: you!

The magic in the mystery is that each cell carries a set of instructions that determines its job. The instructions are written in a blueprint called deoxyribonucleic acid (DNA) for all cells existing or unborn. The genetic code is found in a DNA molecule in every cell of your body. Such coding is a big concept we hear about frequently but do not think about. DNA coding regulates cell life—and thus *your* life. It contains the driving instructions for every cell and body system. It gives each cell one set of rules, tells it what to do, how to live, when to reproduce, and when to die. Every normal cell follows this pattern. In fact, what is common to all cells in all species—and the key to understanding cell mutation in cancer—is the cell's natural life cycle.

Each normal cell has a built-in stop mechanism. In a cancer cell, however, the natural stop mechanism has been turned off (like our out-of-control teenager). Now we have our first clue to the different behavior a cancer cell shows.

We are all living with these cancer cells. Most are identified and expelled from the body, never resulting in traditionally understood cancer. But it's when the body—due to genetic, environmental, behavioral, or unknown reasons—is unable to identify or effectively expel, that is when a particular kind of cancer begins to develop. So how does the body identify these rogue cells? The immune system.*

Before we can proceed, we need a brief but broad understanding of the human immune system. Talk about mysteries! What is the immune system? Where is it? How does it work?—I want to give you a sense of how the body works.† Human beings like other species contain countless communities of cells, but those communities do not welcome strangers. Of course, we need certain bacteria in the stomach, for example. In general, however, the body has to defend itself against internal or external troublemakers like viruses that want to enter to upset the body's balance.

When this happens, the community's defense system—otherwise known as the immune system—comes into play. The immune system stays alert to detect threats, such as harmful bacteria in rotten food or poison from a bug bite, and to identify what it is. Finally, it prescribes solutions to eliminate the threat to community survival.

The immune system has a huge job: to protect the body's integrated communities of cells while they do their work, keeping us alive. The immune system rallies its immune cell army to eliminate invaders much like a police force. Often, the immune system is far ahead of us, inspecting everything going into or leaving the body, and it never stops protecting.

Sometimes though, a potentially harmful cell is not detected or caught by the immune system and it begins to divide randomly, not dying like a normal cell. Now we have a cancer cell without brakes and eventually, a tumor or cluster of cells that competes for resources with other cells making up vital body organs. Unlike viruses or bad bacteria that invade the body, cancer starts with the tiniest part of you . . . a single cell.

---

*For more on this visit www.cancer.gov/cancertopics/understandingcancer/immunesystem/All-Pages.

†Numerous books and online services address general health. For medical topics, go to www.webmd.com.

Survivor Story

When I was young girl I did not know of anyone who had cancer except my grandfather. My grandfather passed away from cancer when my father was eighteen years old. Although I never met my grandfather, I heard stories from my grandmother, my father, and his six brothers and sisters that he was a wonderful hardworking man. My grandfather had a difficult life, away from home for many hours driving a truck, supporting my grandmother and their seven children. While I was growing up my father would speak about my grandfather's brain cancer, how he required surgery, chemotherapy, and radiation, the seizures he would have, and how difficult it was on the family because he was unable to work. In April 1966 at the age of fifty-five my grandfather passed away after battling cancer for two years, never giving up the good fight against a terrible disease. In the 1960s when my grandfather passed away, cancer treatment did not have the technology we have today with computers that assist medical oncologists, surgeons, and radiologists to help them more effectively treat all types of cancer.

I graduated from college in 1999, left my parent's home, and moved to New York City to start a new job. Cancer came back into my life when my thirty-year-old sister, Amy, was diagnosed with a brain tumor. Her illness was diagnosed several months after I started my job. She had just given birth to her third child and we were so excited to have a baby girl in the family. Amy and her husband traveled to several hospitals that specialized in brain tumor treatment. After an extensive search they decided to have the surgery done at Brigham and Women's Hospital in Boston. On January 11, 2000, our family traveled to Boston where she had surgery to remove the cancerous tumor. She went through the regimen of chemotherapy and radiation that was recommended by her doctors. Although she went through the difficulties of cancer treatment, Amy always had a smile on her face and love in her heart for everyone she met.

After two years of battling brain cancer, she passed away at age thirty-two. When this occurred I felt a loss I never experienced in my life. It was so difficult; I was in denial for a long period of time. As my family and I grieved, I tried to search for answers as to why this could happen to my family and her husband and three young children. I was working and trying to do my job and grieving the loss of my sister when I decided to attend a yoga class that was being offered at my job. It was called power vinyasa yoga. I remember the first yoga class and how difficult it was, but more importantly, how it good it made me feel spiritually, mentally, and emotionally. During my first class, my ego kept saying, "You're in great shape, this is nothing," as my legs and arms were trembling.

After this yoga class, I was hooked. I loved how I felt, the freedom of the movement, and the peace I felt after completing the class. I knew this was some-thing I would never stop doing and that it would always be an important part of my life. I became an instructor and I started to teach yoga. The pain and emptiness I felt in my heart because of the death of my sister started to slowly dissipate through my yoga and my teaching. Although my sister was not with me physically, I always felt she was looking over me.

Fast forwarding to 2011, I was living in Las Vegas and still teaching and prac-ticing yoga. I had left my corporate job and I was happy I could start pursuing other interests. My parents came to visit me from Buffalo, New York, and I was ecstatic to be spending time with them. Shortly after they arrived, I started not feeling well with nausea, weakness, and headaches. Although I thought it was the flu, my parents and my boyfriend became increasingly worried because I was not improving after several days.

My mother was in my bedroom taking caring of me when suddenly I had a seizure and lost consciousness for several minutes. My father called 911, the para-medics arrived, and I was rushed to the hospital. I had a head CAT scan done and the ER doctor came in to notify me and my family that I had a six centimeter brain tumor in the left parietal side of my brain. Strangely enough, I was diagnosed with cancer on February 7, 2011, exactly nine years after my sister died on February 7, 2002. The next day I was wheeled into the operating room to have a craniotomy.

When I recovered and came out of surgery, I saw my family and boyfriend by my bedside. I was in disbelief that this could have happened to me. First my dad's father, then Amy, and now me! As I slowly woke up, I was overcome with gratitude to be able to move my fingers and toes, and to be able to breathe. As I began the journey of recovery, I slowly started to do yoga again. At first it was uncomfortable to move, and I focused on my breath and used meditation to help with my fear.

I started radiation and chemotherapy after my surgery and although my body was too tired to move, I kept yoga in my life by meditating and using pranayama. Every day I practiced yoga, even if I could only sit on the bed and do breath-work and arm vinyasas. When I completed my treatments I began to incorporate different movements such as standing poses and seated forward folds. As the weeks progressed, I started to feel stronger. Eight months later, I went back to teaching. As I sat in the classroom looking at my students, I felt every emotion enter my body. I felt an overwhelming sense of gratitude to be able to share this gift of yoga with my students, but more importantly, I had a different apprecia-tion for life and what is truly important. The tribulations of the day when I was diagnosed with brain cancer didn't seem so important, but instead I began to notice the smallest things. This joy that entered my heart has allowed me to *cherish the smallest things and to speak my truth freely. Although I do not know what the future will bring, I know that yoga got me through the darkest days and it will continue to bring me light.*

In the words of Patanjali, "There is always a light within us that is free from all sorrow and grief no matter how much we may be experiencing suffering." This light, I believe, is within me and I hope to share it with all those I encounter.

THE IMMUNE SYSTEM AND HOW IT WORKS

The immune system has many connected components (or subsystems), some of which are discussed here: endocrine, lymphatic, cardiovascular, nervous, musculoskeletal, digestive, respiratory, and skin (integumentary) systems. These may be familiar to us, but less well known is how these different systems work together to create a beautiful symphony of health, defending us from threats by bacteria, viruses, or mutating cells. The immune system has the pivotal job of keeping everything working together so that your body—you—can feel good and enjoy life. Let's take a closer look at how each of these systems work independently and together, providing immunity.

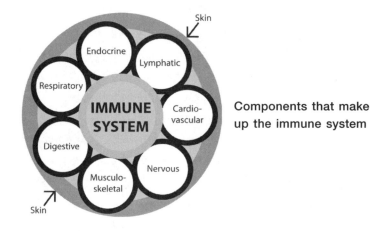

Components that make
up the immune system

Endocrine System

You may be familiar with the fact that the endocrine system produces hormones that tell the body what to do and control how you feel—for example, when you are hungry, sleepy, or fertile. But the endocrine system also makes a hormone in the thymus that links with a white blood cell to form natural, cancer-fighting lymphocytes called T-cells to identify, capture, and kill potential threats.*

---

*Our discussion has to be a general one, although we recognize the many complicated technical questions about how the immune system works on the cellular level.

A virus or bacterium that has caused your flu or cold is easy for the immune system to identify, but cancer is more difficult to detect. Cancer cells do not always look like strangers (which is why I think of them as "sneaky"). Because cancer cells mutate from normal cells, they can escape detection by the body's defenders.

So, the endocrine system has a vital role in the front line of cancer defense. Anti-cancer cells are formed, in effect, with the collaboration of the skeletal system (the bones, where new white blood cells are formed) and the cardiovascular system (the blood that carries our natural, cancer-fighting cells throughout the body to protect us), and they are stored in the lymph nodes, waiting to eliminate mutating cells. All day and night, anti-cancer agents like lymphocytes and T-cells float through the body's blood and lymph fluids on search-and-destroy missions. Most of the time we are well protected.

Lymphatic System

This system is commonly misidentified as encompassing the entire immune system. The lymphatic system provides an infrastructure, starting with a lymph highway—a network of tiny channels that form a one-way passage for lymph fluid to travel throughout the body. This is similar to the cardiovascular system, which consists of veins and arteries that allow blood to circulate. Unlike the cardiovascular system, however, the lymph highway has stopping points and a whole network of "trash bins" called lymph nodes.

A tiny space surrounds most cells, filled with a clear fluid called *interstitial fluid*. Every cell is suspended, waiting in anticipation to be nurtured by a blood supply of proteins, vitamins, hormones, and antibodies. Blood flows into this interstitial fluid to feed and maintain cells. During the process of feeding, cells throw off by-products that are considered waste. This could be anything—dead cells, bacteria, viruses, or other foreign agents.

Suspended in interstitial fluid, debris is then delivered to the lymph system through tiny lymphatic capillaries of the lymph highway, like debris floating down a sewer system on its way to a treatment plant. When the interstitial fluid begins its journey into the lymph system's tiny canals, it is called *lymph fluid*. All day and night, lymph fluid collects throughout the body. In fact, during a normal day in a normal body, four liters of lymph fluid are moved through the body and eliminated.*

---

*For images and information about the thoracic duct, the largest lymphatic vessel, go to www.healthline.com/human-body-maps/thoracic-duct.

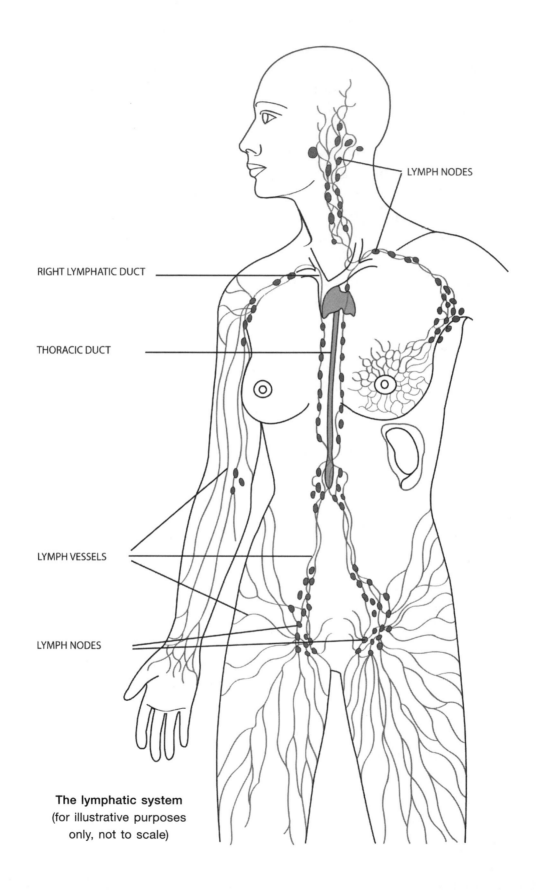

LYMPH NODES

RIGHT LYMPHATIC DUCT

THORACIC DUCT

LYMPH VESSELS

LYMPH NODES

The lymphatic system
(for illustrative purposes
only, not to scale)

Lymph flows through the tiny tunnels connecting nodes, ducts, and glands along the way that serve as containers for examination—the detention centers or reprocessing plants, otherwise known as lymph nodes. Here, the secret agent team of examiners, including lymphocytes and antibodies, wait to sort through the waste for errant cells and toxic elements.

These secret agents will attack rogue cells like cancer once they both arrive in a "detention center." It is here that the T-cells and other disease-fighting agents meet up with the invaders, or mutating cells, from within the body. If, for instance, the right antibody from a flu vaccine is present to neutralize this year's strain, it happens here. The potential threat is irrigated out of the body without causing infection. If it is not, the lymph node or gland enlarges as a sign that there is a "stranger." The virus is isolated while the rest of the immune system rallies assistance. That is why doctors inspect the nodes where they are close to the skin surface, such as under the arms, in the groin, and on the upper chest.

Nodes vary in size and density throughout the body. More of them are located in places like the mouth, nasal passages, and neck, where food and toxins first enter the body. The stomach and intestines are surrounded by lymph glands that are constantly examining waste. In the body's center is the main and most important lymph node—so big it is called a duct. It is here that lymph fluid collects and is conveyed into the venous circulation system to be filtered and flushed out of the body through the spleen, kidneys, liver, and finally, the bladder. The *thoracic duct* is the main detention center of the lymphatic system. It runs parallel to and is nestled close to the spinal column from the top of the lumbar spine (lumbar 2) to the base of the neck (thoracic 1 and cervical 7).

Why do we care? Because the location and function of this duct forms the scientific foundation of yoga's healing power. The thoracic duct along its narrow, long, vertical path is in constant contact with the movement of the horizontal diaphragm muscle, which is massaged by the action of breathing. This knowledge reveals a little secret and creates magic to aid recovery and maintain lifelong health for everyone, not only for the cancer patient and survivor. It is key to the y4c methodology.

Keeping our lymph fluids moving is critical to our health as well, and essential to our immunity. However, unlike the heart of the cardiovascular system, the lymphatic system has no specific muscle. So to cleanse, revitalize, and detoxify our body, the lymphatic system depends on other muscles and gravity to move lymphatic fluids. Here is where I begin to make the case that yoga can be the organ muscle of the lymphatic system. Details on how this works are found in chapter 3, "Benefit 1: Yoga Detoxifies the Body" (page 67–68).

The human body has two fluid highways: blood and lymph. They are similar in structure, but have differences. Lymph has checkpoints along its passageway: nodes, glands, and ducts. We want lymph to stop for examination, but not stay or linger long. On the other hand, we want the blood to flow continuously without interruption.

Cardiovascular System

The meaning of *cardio* is heart. *Vascular* refers to blood vessels, arteries, veins, and capillaries that circulate the blood. Our heart is an organ that pumps oxygenated blood through a vast network of arteries to every part of the body; the deoxygenated blood is circulated back to the heart through our veins. The muscles of the heart create this continuous movement of blood. As blood circulates throughout the body, it carries critical nutrients, antibodies, hormones, enzymes, lymphocytes (our natural anti-cancer agent), and oxygen to all the cells of the body. It also carries away waste products so that they can be removed from the body. Without a blood supply, cells and body tissues would die. The blood always circulates through the body in the same direction.

We all know that keeping blood flowing properly is critical to staying alive. Most everyone is aware that this movement happens best with strong heart muscles and unclogged veins and arteries through which blood can travel. And we are keenly aware of what happens when heart muscles stops or a blood vessel is clogged. The heart is the delivery system of all things good and some things not so good throughout our body. It is an essential team player in the serious business of maintaining immunity.

Nervous System

The nervous system is another line of defense. Receptors in the skin, for example, send nerve signals to the brain with the message, "That stove top is hot!" The nervous system quickly interprets the signal and assesses what could be wrong, sending messages to other systems for help with the threat. In the case of something too hot that would cause a burn, the nervous system tells skeletal muscles to "move away." Such responses have evolved over many millions of years to be extremely rapid and not need conscious thought, which would only slow the response.

Nerves serve as intelligence agents delivering messages to keep information flowing to all parts of the body, and skin and nerves become part of the immune system in the way they work together to identify and analyze danger. Nerves can help to bring about balance, or they can also be a source of false alarm. Too much nervous arousal can be as harmful as too little. There are times when we need stimulation to get systems moving and communicating, as much as we need rest.

Musculoskeletal System

This system is made up of the bones, muscles, cartilage, tendons, ligaments, joints, and other connective tissue that enable our movements and form and protect our internal organs. Its role may seem obvious, but there are hidden gems in it that contribute to our immunity.

Our skeleton not only provides the structure and strength of our body, but it is an essential line of defense. Our bones are so critical to life because they serve as factories for new blood cells. Bone marrow at the center of large bones like the legs and hips is a soft, spongy tissue that produces fresh blood to replenish and maintain all body cells, keeping them alert and functioning so they can protect us from infections and disease.

Muscles are what move the bones. And as they help the body move away from harmful things, this is the obvious role the *musculoskeletal system* plays in the immune system. Nerves, muscles, and bones all work in close concert for even the smallest of actions, like lifting a finger from a hot stove.

However, there is yet another lesser known role. Muscles, small and large, are distributed throughout the body, and aside from moving bones, they also move the soft tissue of organs like the heart, lungs, stomach, and intestines. Internal organs have special muscles to help them function. Inhale, for example, and you're working the diaphragm muscle.

The actions of the muscles in our bowels also demonstrate how healthy muscles are the motors of a healthy immune system. Their job is getting the danger out the door. While all the waste is moving through, something else is happening—a constant analysis and identification of danger by the secret agents that protect us, thanks to the endocrine, lymphatic, and cardiovascular systems. Enzymes, antibodies, and lymphocytes all hang out in our intestines ready to attack threats.

As we move closer to bringing yoga science into this picture, reflect a moment on how collaborative all muscles need to be in order to maintain fully functioning, healthy bodies and keep us out of danger. They work together, whether they are the muscles of your hand moving away from a threatening mosquito about to bite you or respiratory muscles like the diaphragm bringing oxygen to nurture leg muscles when you are taking a walk or running a marathon. Muscle movement is critical to our immunity and well-being.

Digestive System

The digestive system plays an important role in both helping feed the trillion of cells in the body and identifying harmful and foreign toxins. And it's a model of how the body systems are entirely interlinked. For example, that big breakfast you just ate was delicious. Now that you have filled your fuel tank, ready for the hard day ahead, your *digestive system* silently begins to examine everything you ate using tiny muscles to move everything along as it examines and digests the food. Then the digestive system can recognize something harmful, and it activates the muscles to expel what is harmful. It's doing its job when we get sick to our stomach and regurgitate or have diarrhea. Both are a physiological response to a "threat" and it happens with the aid of muscles. Together they play an important part in the immune system.

Respiratory System

Every cell in the body needs a continuous supply of oxygen. That is why we breathe. The respiratory system is designed to move air in and out of our lungs. You might wonder how the respiratory system draws air into the lungs: it starts with the engagement of a special muscle called the diaphragm—a dome-shaped muscle that lies across the bottom of the chest cavity. The diaphragm controls our breathing. With an inhale, it extends downward, making more space for the lungs. With an exhale, it contracts upward to release air out.

When you inhale, air is drawn into the mouth and/or nose, passes through the larynx, trachea, and bronchial tubes, and much like an inflated balloon the lungs expand. The oxygen-rich air fills the nearly 600 million tiny spongy sacs called alveoli. They are surrounded by a network of pulmonary capillaries. Here is where the magic happens. Oxygen is collected and absorbed into the arterial blood stream from the alveoli. At the same time another exchange happens— oxygen-depleted blood flows past the thin walls of the alveoli and releases carbon dioxide into them. This gas exchange—pulling oxygen in and pumping carbon dioxide out—is the primary function of the respiratory system.

However, there is more going on here than the exchange of air and gas. This process removes other unfriendly things besides carbon dioxide from your body. For example, when you inhale through your nose, several things can tickle it, making you sneeze. That is a normal, protective immune response. Your muscles are expelling something identified as foreign, perhaps spring pollen or a cold virus. It's a wonderful response, barring entry into the body before any unwanted element can take hold.

Now let's take this to another level, one of the most magnificent aspects of the human body. How does the respiratory system cultivate immunity and aid our resistance to cancer? Simply, by being the catalyst or electricity to our garbage disposal system—the lymphatic system. The diaphragm's movement assists the lymphatic system by assisting the thoracic duct—the largest lymph node in the body—and its vital role in detoxification. So just like a sneeze, every breath, especially those big ones, helps your body remove harmful foreign bodies, and this includes rogue cancer cells. A thorough explanation of that process is described in chapter 3, Benefit #1: Yoga Detoxifies the Body (pages 67–68).

The wonders of the respiratory system also have a significant impact on both the nervous and cardiovascular systems. Research studies have shown that controlled breathing is an effective relaxation tool that reduces stress hormones, improves sleep, and reduces anxiety. Modifying the pace and depth of our breathing can quiet the mind.[2] Similarly, creating calmness by using simple yoga breathing techniques like *pranayama* (pages 93–94) lowers blood pressure and is a useful tool for those managing cardiovascular disease.[3] We will explore this concept in more detail in Benefit #8: Yoga Helps Manage Fear and Anxiety (pages 75–77).

Skin (Integumentary System)

The skin is a large component of the immune system as well as being the body's largest organ. The skin is our fortress wall, the first line of defense. It covers and protects us, but it also has receptors to send signals through the nervous system when something is potentially dangerous or it senses the presence of something foreign. Think of a sentry flashing a signal to an officer in a tower, asking for a decision.

That is a brief and broad view of how the different systems of the body, working both individually and together, make up the immune system and provide necessary protection. All these are examples of how the body can either identify rogue precancerous cells or support itself to function normally (as in defending against a common cold). It is this basic understanding of human biology that is fundamental to understanding the effectiveness and impact yoga can have on the body and any cancer cells.

In the next section we will explore scientific principles of physics and anatomy that demonstrate how yoga can support these systems and functions. Even the science of psychology, in which consciousness and emotions are studied, can be applied to yoga practices of meditation and mindfulness. Let's take a closer look at the science behind the practice of yoga and begin to address how yoga can help in the healing process, improve risk factors, and make you feel better.

SCIENTIFIC FOUNDATION
OF THE Y4C METHODOLOGY

Yoga is as scientific as it is spiritual. Laws of physics like gravity govern the body and its movement in the same way they govern machines' functions. Yoga follows principles of movement, resistance and restriction of movement, gravity, and the relaxation response. In addition, yoga's spiritual benefits can be explained through research from psychology, something you don't usually hear about in yoga class. Powerful ideas from physics, biology, and psychology provide the science behind yoga to keep the body and mind clear, balanced, and strong.

WHY MOVEMENT IS IMPORTANT

We need to understand motion, how it works, and the value of movement at all stages of life. Perhaps the greatest strength of yoga is that all muscles, bones, and body systems are stimulated to promote health. Yoga focuses each of us on the mechanics of movement, and to keep the body healthy, several kinds of movement are needed. After all, movement is our daily companion, whether it is transferring the whole body from place to place, or moving parts to accomplish life's tasks like combing your hair or using a keyboard. Many more unseen types of movement occur under the skin without conscious direction, like the circulation of oxygen to the cells or the movement of food through the digestive tract.

The body is built to move! The human body is continuously both growing and decaying. Our bones, for instance, are losing mass and being rebuilt at the same time that old cells are dying and new ones are being born. Without movement, decay occurs faster than growth, and the body begins to break down.[4] For instance, extended bed rest causes muscles to atrophy and bones to thin. Movement helps to keep body systems in a state of balance. Even not moving involves movement. Just balancing the body requires the muscular movement of extension and contraction. We are, of course, usually not aware of the constant subtle adjustments our muscles make to simply sit in a chair or stand in one spot on two feet, much less find balance in a handstand.

The right kind of movement builds both strength and flexibility! Moving our muscles maintains and improves strength and flexibility that allows us to perform the activities of daily living (ADLs) essential to quality of life. The ability to bend down and tie a shoe, to carry home groceries, and to put food away on a top shelf without pain, discomfort, or exhaustion—all are forms of independence we may not consider until we encounter the physical challenges that can come with surgery, illness, inactivity, or old age.

EXERCISE IS MEDICINE

"Exercise is medicine," says Dr. Andrea Cheville, associate professor of physical medicine and rehabilitation at the Mayo Clinic.* Two thousand years ago, the ancient Greek physician Hippocrates advanced the *rest theory* to cure disease. In the past one hundred years, exercise was only seen as preventive to disease. Only recently in the last twenty-five years has exercise been studied for its proactive healing and life-extending potential.†

Today, the importance of movement for health is more acknowledged than in the past. Increasingly, the value of movement over rest has been recognized for serious diseases like diabetes, arthritis, asthma, hypertension, and cancer. The American Cancer Society recommends 150 minutes of moderate activity or seventy-five minutes of strenuous activity for healthy adults spread throughout the week to reduce the risk of cancer, cardiovascular disease, and diabetes.‡ The well-known physician Dean Ornish benchmarked the use of exercise to prevent and manage heart disease, and he created a program designed to reverse heart disease.[5]

Other studies support the value of movement and exercise for healing. A 2001 study of more than 116,000 women found that exercise reduces mortality.[6] A 2005 study at Brigham and Women's Hospital in Boston linked exercise to cancer recovery during and after breast cancer treatments. They found that exercise reduced common side effects and enhanced mood. This study measured how, over time, three to four hours of walking per week can reduce the risk of breast cancer-related death by 50 percent.[7]

"The leap has been made," according to Jörg Blech in his book, *Healing through Exercise*, "Move, move, move in order to overcome illness and lengthen your life."[8] But the understandable recommendation by health professionals

---

*The work of Dr. Andrea Cheville is presented by Mona Kleinberg in "Working It Out: Exercise and Weight Management for Health and Well-Being," *Insight*, Spring (2006): 1. *Insight* is a quarterly publication of Living Beyond Breast Cancer (www.lbbc.org/About-LBBC).

†For more information about Hippocrates, see http://en.wikipedia.org/wiki/Hippocrates. For general discussion of the growing case for exercise and cancer, see Jörg Blech, *Healing through Exercise* (New York: Merloyd Lawrence Books/Perseus, 2009), chapter 12.

‡The American Cancer Society has recommendations for reducing the risk of cancer as well as helpful tools for assessing health: www.cancer.org/healthy/index.

to cancer patients after the surgeries, chemotherapy, and radiation treatments has been, "Go home and take it easy." Although exercise is gaining favor as a recommendation for recovery, I worry that health care professionals who found it easier to write a prescription for a drug will only send patients to a fitness specialist in the hospital's complementary clinic, or refer them to the local gym, the source of clinically-controllable traditional methods that have been used in studies over the past twenty-five years: walking on a treadmill, jogging, and weight training. Eastern spiritual practices like yoga or t'ai chi have been less studied, so they are not as likely to be recommended.

Current research fails to explain *how* and *why* exercise prolongs life, speeds recovery, or improves quality of life, only that it does. These studies are based on easily measurable outcomes from walking, jogging, and weight lifting. Why not study the effects of yoga, qigong, and t'ai chi like Ornish did with his cardiac patients in 1985? The success of these studies on exercise and cancer will encourage research to continue. As a result, we will learn more about the ways that exercise seems to protect the body. The challenge for researchers, clinicians, and the Western medical community is to figure out which types of exercise work best. A recent review of the literature on yoga and cancer found support for increased well-being but pointed to a difficult challenge for researchers—the need for better theory.[9] One of the hard problems for researchers is isolating the components within a complex activity like yoga that are most effective for certain people and specific cancers.

Survivor Story

Thank God for yoga.

The key was finding the right class. As an experienced yogi, I wanted to continue my vinyasa practice but after a mastectomy with lymph nodes removed and rounds of chemo and radiation, it was impossible. I continued my practice throughout it all. I taught athletic yoga. I got a nosebleed once from showing off in a headstand during chemo, which was not fun. When I lost my hair, students just thought it was a Buddhist thing or some such devotional side effect.

My classes boomed.

Finding Tari's class was an eye-opener. I finally felt at ease with a teacher who knew my situation. My left arm tingled and my chest was tight with ribs broken. I was worried about lymphedema. She really knew her stuff and I felt safe. She hit all the right points and in such a loving, kind, and knowledgeable way. I was home.

The cancer spread to my sternum and I had 40 percent of it removed, which was painful but effective. Wheel pose is no longer an option, try as I might. It is hard to see my abilities diminish but my understanding of true yoga has deepened. It's not just about a pretty pose. It's the ability to be in the moment completely.

Letting go.

The cancer spread again, stage 4 with bone metastasis in the hips and spine. My hips are now arthritic, a side effect from my radiation and inflammation. Mary, a teacher, showed me some wonderfully gentle hip openers that literally began to take down the swelling. I teach it to my classes now. Cancer recently returned to my spine and I've just finished a third round of radiation. The vertebrae are so fragile, I was told no lifting, no yoga, no anything! Brace time! So say the surgeons. This is where the real yoga happens.

A strong yet gentle practice is how I am surviving. When asked by the doctors how I support my spine, I tell them, "with my core." If that were weak, my back would break. Aside from the strength, yoga keeps me focused. It allows me to flow and breathe and stretch out all the sadness, the fear, and the anxiety. I see it, I flow with it, and I let it go. But I do feel it. You must in order to let it go. Yoga teaches you that. Taking the practice off the mat and applying it to life is a beautiful thing. It's not always easy but I have noticed since all of this cancer and terror and uncertainty, it has become crucial. Also, it just happened, without me even noticing.

For some of us, cancer is like a fast pass to enlightenment. I understand so much more than I did before all of this happened. It has made me a better teacher. I see my young, healthy students during classes, checking pedicures, peeking at messages on their iPhones—no clue. Take a look at the students in a yoga class. Ideally they are all completely and beautifully focused. Our life, or quality of life, depends on it. It is important. It is amazing.

The relaxation and meditation periods are stronger now. Without deep relaxation, we don't heal. It's a fact. I am able to sit still and listen to my body, to my breath, or to nothing at all. The ability to clear the mind to make room for what's important is huge for me. Cancer puts you into a state of chaos and shock. I can't find anything and it's not just due to chemo brain or hormone suppressants, it's stress related.

I have lost much to cancer. Aside from the obvious body parts—breasts, lymph nodes, thyroid, sternum, hair (grew back), eyelashes (still missing)—there are deeper losses. People: partners, friends, and even family have slowly disappeared from my life. It's too much for them to handle. Gone are all the things I thought were needed for a "normal" life. In its place I have found a new under-standing of true friendship—with myself and others.

Yoga teaches me to practice vairagya, *or nonattachment. To not be attached is key. It is paired with* abhyasa, *practice. When everything outside is gone, what is left? That is the yoga.*

The right yoga practice is everything.

WHAT HAPPENS WHEN WE MOVE?

When we move, the heart beats, body fluids flow, and breathing increases. When we exercise and when we practice active yoga poses or sequences, we are engaging our skeletal muscles. Contracting muscles consumes large amounts of oxygen. Because oxygen and nutrients are delivered to our muscles through the blood, this causes the heart to pump faster and our circulation to increase in order to support the meta-bolic and contractile activity of the muscles. Exercising cardiac muscle makes it both stronger and more efficient, improving cardiovascular health. Increased circulation also aids the movement of lymphatic fluid throughout the body.

Regular exercise improves health as well as mental well-being.[10] Yoga is exer-cise, of course, but how does it work, and in what ways does yoga benefit us? Forms of physical exercise such as yoga appear to improve thinking due to increased blood and oxygen flow to the brain, and increased levels of neurotransmitters like endor-phins, especially dopamine, that improve mood and thus aid motivation.[11]

HOW DO WE MOVE?

Motion is simply a change in position. Staying healthy involves moving two things: our bones and essential body fluids. There are several kinds of body movement to consider if we want to understand how yoga works, and the physiology and phys-ics behind the y4c methodology. These movements include *stretching (flexion* and *extension), expanding* and *contracting, twisting, squeezing, soaking,* and *resistance.*

Movement happens when muscles alternate between flexion and exten-sion—the bending or unbending of joints or limbs. To lift an arm bone, move blood through the channels of veins, or draw air into our lungs—muscles exert their effects through a lattice-like fan of fibers, expanding and contract-ing. A muscle is body tissue designed to stretch, contract, squeeze, twist, and activate other parts of the body.

The first of these actions, stretching—the best-known yoga movement—is the effort to make space between two points, as in moving point A away from point B. When you stretch a muscle, you are trying to lengthen it by working it in two directions simultaneously.

The opposite movement of shortening that space is called *contracting*. Expanding and contracting are really part of the same movement because in order to expand one set of muscles, another set must contract. It is the alternation of these two actions that creates stretching. For example, when you fold your fingers into a fist, the muscles on the back of your hand lengthen. When you stretch the fingers open, the opposite happens—the muscles in your palm extend, while the muscles on the back of the hand contract.

The action of twisting is similar to stretching because the goal is to create space between two points. What makes twisting different is that it is a spiral around an axis. For example, pulling the right shoulder away from the left hip in a rotational-type movement creates a spinal twist. The spine must be held properly upright.

Muscles also squeeze, using the same expand-and-contract action with one difference: action occurs in one direction at a time. Consider the muscles that are designed to assist organs to function, such as the heart or intestines. When stimulated, these muscles first become shorter by contracting inward. Then the opposite happens and they release, expanding or lengthening outward. When this action happens around the soft tissue of organs, movement of fluid is produced. For example, when your heart beats, the heart muscle is contracting inward, which pushes blood out of the heart into the arteries. The opposite movement of releasing the same muscle draws blood back and creates a soaking action. In the action of squeezing, muscles move toward a single point; in soaking, muscles move away from a single point.

SQUEEZE-AND-SOAK EFFECT

The phrase *squeeze and soak* was coined by B. K. S. Iyengar to describe the process in which poses such as yoga twists create physical compression and affect fluid circulation.[12] Iyengar taught that twists cleanse our internal organs in the same way that a sponge discharges dirty water when squeezed and can then absorb fresh water and expand. Blood is squeezed out of the affected area and, as compression is released, the area is soaked with fresh, oxygenated blood to fuel healthy organs and muscles. The health claims of the squeeze-and-soak action in relationship to blood circulation have not been established. However, lymphatic flow can be improved by compression. Massage therapy and compression stockings are common methods used to successfully aid lymphatic drainage, using the principles of compression.

RESISTING MOVEMENT: RESTRICTION

The same muscular efforts of extension and flexion, when combined with a specific opposing force, create resistance. Resistance is movement against an opposing force, such as a wall, the floor, a table, or even gravity. In fact, the body is resisting gravitational force all the time, awake or asleep, in walking, running, or sitting. We may not think about gravity very much, but muscles and bones have evolved to help us cope with and depend upon it. As we will learn, yoga utilizes the force of gravity to strengthen bones and muscles.

In the science of physics and yoga, holding the body in stillness—resisting movement—can require as much muscular effort as propelling the body into motion. There are two kinds of resistance effort: *active* and *passive*. An example of active resistance would be holding a standing pose for a length of time, or for several breath counts. In this situation, muscular effort maintains the pose along with the acts of stretching, twisting, and breathing. The body is still, yet muscles are working.

An example of passive resistance would be removing muscular effort and allowing the force of gravity to hold the body in a stretch or twisting pose—a fundamental concept in restorative yoga.

A less familiar, but powerful, technique is to use an external force, such as a strategically placed hand, yoga strap, or weight, to assist creating an inwardly-directed squeezing force. The goal is to gently guide body fluids in a specific direction. This technique is used successfully in lymphatic massage therapy to manage conditions like lymphedema. Compression garments like compression sleeves and stockings also create a similar, yet passive, force.

MYSTERIES OF YOGA
UNVEILED BY BIOLOGY

Everyone knows yoga is "good for you," but not everyone knows why. The common assumption is that yoga is a great relaxation technique or a fabulous way to get a good muscle stretch. Looking deeper into the biology of the human body, there are other important ways yoga is good for us. Lymphatic drainage, venous return, and bone building are not as commonly associated with yoga but are important biological functions in pursuit of good health. Understanding how the human body works and how yoga helps to make it work better, easier, and more efficiently is the beginning of a healthy partnership and unveils some of the mysteries of yoga as well as our body.

When our body fluids (blood and lymph) are flowing properly, we strengthen our immune system and aid expulsion of waste and potentially harmful toxins. Lymphatic drainage and venous return are two important body functions that keep things flowing using the natural tools of muscle movement and gravity. Yoga can assist.

Survivor Story

Cancer caused me more suffering than anything I ever experienced, and I was able to relieve some of the pain through yoga. As a longtime survivor of HIV, I had known illness but I was not prepared for the agony of cancer. When I was diagnosed with Hodgkin's lymphoma in November, 2009, I was already heavily involved with yoga. I had been practicing for ten years and I had a place in the yoga community. I had a teacher who instilled her voice within me. I attended public classes and I had a home practice. I was even a volunteer yoga teacher for people with HIV and other life-threatening illnesses. My partner, Michael, was in a yoga teacher training program through most of my illness. His support, strengthened by his own yoga immersion, helped save my life.

Yoga was a place to go during my illness. In a life scheduled with doctor's appointments and chemotherapy, yoga became something "normal" scheduled into my day. It was something to do besides having cancer.

A friend and yoga teacher gave me a restorative practice that was supposedly handed down from Iyengar himself. I practiced yoga at least four times a week during my illness. Cancer tried to take yoga away from me. It robbed me of most of my physical strength and it cut to the heart of my yoga practice by trying to rob me of my breath. I was able to persevere. Yoga was a way to reclaim some energy and it was an opportunity to turn my attention away from the outer world—a world now lived in hospitals and infusion rooms. Yoga gave me a way to quiet my mind. Through yoga I was able to stay somewhat connected to a body that was always in pain.

Two weeks after I finished chemotherapy my partner was diagnosed with prostate cancer. His diagnosis forced the battle onward at a time when we were both already exhausted from the war. In a matter of weeks and then over the following months the patient had to immediately become the caretaker. As my own body began to heal, my yoga practice became more energized. Yoga provided some relief from the anxiety of these times. I returned to public classes and reconnected with yoga friends and yoga teachers, who became part of my support network.

The ending was happy. We both survived and our relationship survived. Yoga gave me a significant part of what I needed to battle my own cancer and then it provided me with the strength to persist through my partner's cancer. Yoga kept me hopeful and eased my fears through the most difficult journey of my life. Yoga was one of the few constants during a time when everything changed.

Lymphatic Drainage

Unlike our cardiovascular system, our lymphatic system does not have a pump to move the four liters of lymph fluid daily through the body. Consequently, the lymphatic system depends on physical movement and gravity to keep things flowing or prevent build up of unwanted waste (toxins, cells, or other waste). Lymphatic drainage is the continuous one-directional movement of lymph fluid from all parts of our body through the lymph channels toward the thoracic duct, the principle cleansing station of our body. This drainage process is created by several different kinds of movement.

Internal movement
- Contraction and flexion of muscles moves our bones
- Muscle compression creates the squeeze-and-soak effect (see page 49)
- Increased heart rate moves blood, lymph fluid, and breath
- Breathing moves the diaphragm and massages the thoracic duct (see pages 67–68)

External movement
- The natural pull of gravity
- Lymphatic massage or brushing*

Yoga is designed to assist these natural movements and body functions to aid the detoxification of the body.[†]

---

*Lymphatic massage is a technique developed in Germany for treatment of lymphedema, an accumulation of lymph fluid that can occur after lymph nodes are removed. Because the lymph nodes and channels are close to the skin, this simple, gentle technique is a manual directional movement to follow the lymphatic channels and designed to increase flow of lymph fluid. See M. Foldi and R. Strobenreuther, *Foundations of Manual Lymph Drainage*, Elseuier Mosby Press, 2003.

[†]For more on lymphedema and how yoga can help see www.breastcancer.org/treatment/lymphedema/how/lymph_system and yogainternational.com/article/view/5-natural-ways-to-relieve-lymphatic-congestion.

Venous Return

The heart pumps oxygenated blood through our arteries to every part of the body and pulls deoxygenated blood back to the heart through our veins. When we are in an upright position, deoxygenated blood must travel upward through our veins from our lower body to return to the heart. This is venous return. Like water being pumped uphill through a hose, the venous return of our blood is slowed by the pull of gravity. Extended inactivity can cause blood to pool in the legs, potentially causing swelling, blood clots, and varicose veins. Yoga inversions like a headstand use gravity to help aid venous return to the heart from the lower body and more efficient recirculation of oxygenated blood.

Bone Building

Resistance against the pull of gravity puts stress on our bones, which is needed to keep them strong. Osteoblasts and osteoclasts are the specialized bone cells responsible for bone mass. Osteoblasts produce bone matrix, resulting in increased bone mass. Osteoclasts reabsorb bone matrix, resulting in decreased bone mass. Osteoblasts and osteoclasts maintain a dynamic balance in response to the mechanical needs of the bones. Just as movement increases muscle strength, resistance against gravity increases the activity of osteoblasts and strengthens bones. So yoga poses that involve weight bearing on the bones, such as standing and balancing poses, increase the active resistance of our bones against gravity, improving bone health.

RELAXATION RESPONSE

The most commonly expected benefit of yoga—relaxation—cannot be underestimated or undervalued. The biomechanical and biochemical benefits of relaxation are well researched and universally experienced. The chronic stress of daily life can over-activate the sympathetic nervous system, potentially causing a wide range of effects including high blood pressure, headaches, fatigue, insomnia, anxiety, and depression. In the 1960s, Dr. Herbert Benson of Harvard Medical School proved that the brain can be stimulated to create relaxation.[13] He called this the *relaxation response* and described it as a physical state of deep rest that changes our physical and emotional responses to stress. Relaxation occurs when the parasympathetic nervous system is activated.

There is no single method for eliciting the relaxation response; however, practices like the following are recommended: slow breathing, focusing the mind, and relaxing muscle tension. Meditation and restorative yoga poses can be effective.

Active yoga poses also may be practiced with these three principles in mind to create a relaxation response while also offering all the health benefits of movement.

Before we consider additional insights from the field of psychology, let's review some of the scientific principles of yoga. First, physics is at work on the biomechanics of the body when we do yoga. Second, this activity directly affects our biology on a cellular level. Finally, together these foundations form the scientific explanation of how yoga works to assist the immune system in its job of protecting the body and decreasing the risk of cancer.

I believe long-term hope and health begin with studying the body and mind while building a personal yoga practice to improve well-being and reduce risk of cancer (and other challenges of aging). After all, human beings are resilient and cancer can be a motivating factor in learning about the body and health. Most cancers can be managed for years if caught early, and we use the threat to our advantage by monitoring what we eat, how we exercise, and how we manage stress. Facing danger, we evaluate what is most important in life.

Earlier we discussed a cell's natural life cycle and the fact that each normal cell has a built-in stop mechanism, unlike a cancer cell that behaves like an out-of-control teenager. The body needs new cells and produces countless generations of new cells throughout life. Many types of cancer-fighting cells, such as T-cells, are also produced by the body. Much of the new learning we are cultivating is at the cellular and molecular level, which are not topics discussed in yoga texts or in classes.

The body protects us most of the time and this critical work needs a strong immune system that keeps blood fresh, clean, and rich with life-giving oxygen and healing nutrients. The body is protected by the immune system's layered defenses against threats like rogue cells through the efforts of several systems of the body. The lymphatic system, in particular, provides a lymph highway to move toxins and precancerous cells from the body. And we have discussed how yoga improves health, since yoga poses and deep breathing stimulate lymph drainage, using principles of physics, gravity, and purposeful body movement.

Finally, research from every discipline says that regular exercise improves physical health as well as mental well-being. To recover and then stay healthy, each day we seek ways to move and thus strengthen three things: bones, muscles, and essential body fluids like blood and lymph. Structured poses and yoga sequences build our bones and muscles and, just as importantly, move blood and lymph fluids to protect us. The mechanics of movement in yoga poses stimulate muscles, bones, and body systems to promote health.

PSYCHOLOGY AND YOGA

Powerful insights about yoga and its benefits have come from cognitive social psychology and counseling psychology. Another relevant area is positive psychology, a field developed in the last thirty years by Martin Seligman and his colleagues that focuses on personal growth and development rather than life's problems. The emphasis on positive self-evaluation is akin to what yoga calls *maitri,* or loving kindness to self and compassion toward others.

People are not asked to ignore or deny challenges like cancer or any stressful situation, but to think about how to manage the challenge. We control what we can while acknowledging that many things in life are beyond our control. The dominant model of psychotherapy today, cognitive behavioral therapy, focuses people on how they think and behave more than on deep motives or personality traits that had interested therapists in the last century.

A large body of research is building on mindfulness. Some mindfulness experts like Jon Kabat-Zinn focus on meditation, health, and the spiritual aspects of mindfulness, while others like Ellen Langer focus on how people think about life, asking us to challenge our biases and errant mindsets—and to pay attention to the present moment. Much more is known today about techniques for relaxation to lower anxiety or improve health, like different forms of meditation or a specific method like guided imagery, in which people are asked to imagine themselves visiting different parts of the body.*

Psychologist Robert Ader and immunologist Nicholas Cohen have created a field called psychoneuroimmunology.[14] Their creative research mapped the body's communication network among immune cells, hormones, and neurotransmitters. Their work explored the science behind ideas once considered superstitious: that meditation reduces arterial plaque; that social bonds improve cancer survival; that people under stress catch more colds; and that placebos work not only on the human mind but also on individual cells. Their innovative research also supports the theory that stress on the nervous system worsens illness—and perhaps even causes it—and that reducing stress is vital to health.†

---

*For more about relaxation, go to http://jnci.oxfordjournals.org/content/94/8/558.short.
†Scientists measure stress by changes in cortisol levels in the body. Also, it is the extremes of stress—too high or too low—or rapid changes in level that are harmful to the body.

PERSONALITY TRAITS,
PERSONAL BELIEFS, AND CANCER

A cancer diagnosis for most people is upsetting. "How could this have happened to me?" we ask. At such times, some people are tempted to blame themselves, which then only adds to the stress. A few decades ago it was asserted (without much evidence) that a type C personality increased vulnerability (the supposed trait was loosely defined by introversion, conflict avoidance, and perfectionism). Some yoga practitioners still use this outdated notion that is not helpful.

A personality theory of cancer is tempting but wrong. While it is true that choices we make in life like smoking, drinking too much alcohol, or not controlling our weight are risk factors, these are not personality factors. Even then, it takes a chance mutation of an errant cell and an immune system that does not catch that cell to spark the possible cancer.

The American Cancer Society reviews studies of personality traits and cancer—and no evidence has been found that a personality trait or a particular attitude or belief plays any role in getting cancer or surviving it.[15] Having a positive attitude helps people keep going and psychotherapy can provide support to improve quality of life—but the evidence today is that neither increase survival. However, improved quality of life and a long survivorship—although they are not the same—are both important outcomes and goals of any healthy pursuit we undertake, like yoga.

LEARNING IN GROUPS

Although this book is about providing you with the necessary knowledge and tools to develop a home practice, I do not want you to underestimate the role of a yoga class or group. One of the unspoken secrets of cancer is the loneliness it creates. You feel this is happening only to you. Cancer patients find themselves in distracted states of mind, bombarded with frightening facts, and subjected to invasive procedures in cold clinical environments. A yoga class for survivors can be the one safe environment that quiets the mind and restores the body. And it can be a place to witness how others are living with fear. I tell my yoga students, "Don't do it alone. Learning from others makes us stronger."

Human beings make meaning of their lives in every setting, and a yoga community is an excellent place for this work. Research in the social and health sciences supports the benefits of social groups for health and well-being, especially when facing a challenge like cancer. Facing such a challenge on your own is difficult because motivation may be low to stay with treatment schedules, causing stress that ultimately results in reduced healing. You do not want to be alone in this fight!

People respond to their social and physical environments, often in unseen and unknown ways. If, for instance, we want to change a personal behavior, like getting more exercise, it is hard to do this by yourself. It's better to change the peer groups and environmental cues that supported the old behavior.[16] This notion would suggest that strengthening your body is more likely if you ask a friend to go for a walk, join a social group that exercises, or find a yoga class led by a yoga teacher knowledgeable of the risks, needs, and desires of cancer patients.

ALTERNATIVE MEDICINE AND THE PLACEBO EFFECT

Fifty years of personality and social psychology research underscore the power of the expectations people set for themselves (and others), including responses to cancer treatment and the way they approach yoga. People are asked to set clear, positive goals, have reasonable expectations, be curious, focus on the process of learning more than the results, and remain willing to revise the plan.

The expectations we hold for these therapies and medicines are a serious problem for research that tries to separate true causes from all the claims made in the marketplace about cures. Yoga is part of the expanding field of complementary and alternative medicine (CAM), and the federal government is now providing financial support for research.* While evidence is growing that yoga or acupuncture can reduce stress and promote well-being, that is not the same as preventing molecular diseases like cancer, or increasing survival. Again, individuals may be helped or feel better because of a placebo response. But this does not justify the widespread use of a particular remedy or type of therapy. Impassioned testimonials often drive the popularity of an unproven or alternative therapy, but Western science sets a high standard.

---

*Alternative medicine refers to substitutions for traditional medicine, whereas complementary medicine integrates mainstream medicine and alternative methods. The National Institutes of Health has a division to focus on best practices and new research in complementary and alternative medicine called the National Center for Complementary and Alternative Medicine (NCCAM). See http://nccam.nih.gov/.

The gold standard for empirical proof in Western science is the randomized control trial (RCT), sometimes called a prospective study, which is a stringent test of validity using numbers, not feelings and testimonials. The problem is that expectations for the desired effect, often unconscious, are powerful in both healing and in contaminating research. So, in Western research, both experimenters and the people they study have to be kept "blind" for the purpose of the research, or the experimenter risks the powerful placebo effect in which participants anticipate what is wanted and provide it to the experimenter.

The goal is, after all, to find a therapy or remedy in the right dose that works reliably for all or most people, not just for the one person who believes that this or that vitamin or type of massage is curative. Again, individual well-being may benefit, which is fine—but that is not the same standard as a proven cure. Paul Offit makes this point in his book with the provocative title, *Do You Believe in Magic: The Sense and Nonsense of Alternative Medicine.* He finds little scientific support for most dietary supplements and alternative healing strategies.[17] It is not hard in this day and age to find charlatans, Offit says, who claim their "new" machine or "miracle" supplement cures cancer, when careful research finds the claims self-serving, erroneous, and even harmful to people who may then avoid chemotherapy or other effective treatments. Why are people so vulnerable to these false claims? Offit says that mainstream doctors appear distant, uncaring, and just "too busy," prescribing feared surgeries and regimens like chemotherapy. Alternative practitioners can seem empathic and compassionate, have more time for patients and families, and provide "natural" remedies that are less scary.* Survivors want to find hope and can be vulnerable to unproven claims, especially when the cancer is advanced and according to Western medicine there is little more that can be done to help them. Offit has fun debunking the many hoaxes in the field of alternative medicine, but he has a serious and good motive: he wants mainstream medicine to appreciate the best alternative strategies, in particular, placebo responses that improve well-being, and alternative medicine to understand the limits of their methods for dangerous, complex diseases like metastatic cancer.

Researchers have worried about the placebo effect for many years because

---

*Offit also argues that alternative cures that are expensive contribute to a well-documented cognitive effect in social psychology called *dissonance reduction.* In effect, we ask, "Why am I paying so much for this? It must be great!"

it contaminates research. Offit's view is different and creative; he embraces the placebo response. While the explanations or theory for improvement are deceptive and wrong, some people do get relief. More importantly, the body can learn to produce endorphins in response to expectations of being helped, a critical mind-body connection.

Finally, the placebo effect is one of the most important and complex mind-body phenomena, and I believe we have just begun to disentangle effects and causal directions. We just do not know enough yet about most CAM therapies. Claims are made but rigorous empirical research is in its infancy.

DOES YOGA
REDUCE CANCER RISK?

Does a regular yoga practice reduce the possibility of getting cancer in the first place, or help get rid of active tumors? Readers may have this hard question in mind, and the answer is not simple. Both research and personal experience lead me to believe that yoga strengthens the immune system, increases well-being and sense of personal control, and reduces cancer risk. That is why I have given my life to y4c. We reduce risk and improve the odds, but still have no guarantee.

Cancer involves so many factors. We have many things to learn! We do not understand, for instance, what turns off the immune system or turns it back on. How do some errant cells get through the layered defenses when most of the time the multiple defenses work well for us? We are learning more and more about the highly individualized nature of most cancers, which points to new interventions that tailor treatment of individual tumors and mutating cells at the genetic level. But does that mean that every intervention has to be unique and thus costly? How will these costs be funded as cancer incidence increases? The public health dilemmas are profound.

The ancient wisdom of yoga finds support in the research and careful logic of modern science. Yoga is not at odds with Western medicine even though medical language can sound strange (yoga terms are unusual too). It requires thinking like a scientist to understand the body and its biomechanics, and to explore puzzles about how the mind and the body work. Both Eastern and Western ways of knowing have much to give us, but the gifts are quite different. We need both.

Preventing cancer is a difficult issue because empirical research of the effects of yoga on cancer has only begun. We do not know enough yet about causes or the biology of cancer to try to answer all questions with the methods we have today. But we have to try.

Many research studies point to the positive benefits of yoga in coping with fatigue, insomnia, depression, and anxiety, and improving quality of life—and all this is valuable.* Yoga is recommended by medical authorities in an integrative approach that includes the best Western approaches, even if some treatments like chemotherapy will be judged as quite primitive a hundred years from now. Still, the American Cancer Society remains cautious, saying as yet no scientific evidence exists that yoga prevents cancer in a specific individual, or increases survival.

We do know that smoking, lack of exercise, and being overweight increase cancer risk, and chronic stress may also be a risk factor. A recent study from the American Association for Cancer Research reported that postmenopausal women who walk an hour a day can reduce their chance of developing breast cancer.[18] A yoga practice can help you feel more in control of your life, which might lead you to better choices about diet and other habits. And I have argued that a strong immune system that results from a regular yoga practice will increase quality of life and aid recovery while reducing risk of cancer and other serious disease.

Finally, when learning to manage your recovery and working on your personal wellness plan, some risk taking is better than being too passive when it comes to a new interest like yoga. While some cancer treatments require us to be careful, people benefit from a daily routine of movement and meditation like yoga offers.

Yoga with a trained teacher works to strengthen all major body systems, especially the immune system. Stronger muscles and bones result along with increased flexibility. We begin to see how the mind works and learn how to use the breath and meditation to control anxiety and depression, thus improving concentration and allowing us be productive at whatever we choose to do. Yoga is a tested discipline, centuries old, that encourages and rewards self-control. And most people learn yoga in the community of others, which also brings benefits to health and well-being. What other system of exercise offers so much?

---

*For example, a recent meta-analysis of thirteen prospective studies, mostly of breast cancer, found large beneficial effects of yoga in reducing distress, anxiety, and depression; moderate beneficial effects on fatigue, general health-related quality of life, emotional function, and social function; and insignificant effect on sleep (Buffart et al, "Physical and Psychosocial Benefits of Yoga in Cancer Patients," www.biomedcentral.com/1471-2407/12/559).

Core ingredients and benefits of yoga are increasingly supported by both Western and Eastern medical thinking. In the chapters ahead, you'll read about how yoga poses and movements to increase physical and emotional strength are supported by medicine. Now we'll turn to the language of yoga. The goal is to create a new narrative or life story for yourself that's scientifically based out of the challenge of cancer, and to find a positive, fulfilling yoga practice that allows you to control as much of your life as possible.

Survivor Story

I was diagnosed with breast cancer in April 2013, and two months later I had a left-side mastectomy and tissue expander followed by chemotherapy, which I finished in January 2014. My original plastic surgeon was fundamentally opposed to most forms of upper-body exercise, and the little that I was "permitted" to do was revealed only after I pried it out of him and his staff; it was never suggested to me. They did not tell me about many things, including the existence of an exercise program at the same hospital, but by a stroke of luck I heard about it and attended an information day at the hospital. One of the presenters was someone who led an exercise class for breast cancer survivors, and at this class I learned about Tari's y4c classes.

When I was finished with my chemo I wanted to resume some modified forms of exercise. I had exercised almost every day for years before my cancer diagnosis but only had the energy for some easy lower-body cardio throughout the chemo treatments. I tried to go back to the intermediate vinyasa yoga classes I had been taking before my surgery, avoiding most upper-body weight bearing as per the doctor. However I underestimated how weak the surgery side was, even though I was being very cautious, and somehow got a small muscle tear in my back. Then I remembered the y4c classes, and tried my first one in February 2014.

Tari leads the students in a class that resembles the kind of yoga I used to do, but it is safer and takes into account the osteopenia that I and other women have as a result of chemotherapy or age. Also, I was able to switch to the care of a new, more enlightened surgeon who advocates exercise (and who said that the osteopenia may have been partially from not exercising for so long). Some of that couldn't be helped due to the chemo but mostly it was due to the restrictions from the original surgeon.

I am so grateful to Tari for giving me back my yoga practice!

*Nothing will work
unless you do.*

MAYA ANGELOU

Deborah, cancer survivor

3

Applying the Science for Recovery and Prevention

We turn now to the specific benefits of yoga for those touched by cancer. Chapter 2 provided a basic understanding of the physics, biology, and psychology of both yoga and cancer. This chapter applies these foundations and provides specific research to demonstrate how a yoga practice supports the healing process and should be part of every person's wellness plan. Below is an example of an interaction I had with a student that demonstrates the empathetic role of the yoga teacher and the types of challenges a cancer survivor faces.

"Is this the yoga for cancer class?" the woman asked, having placed her mat on the floor. She seemed unsure of her surroundings, like most women who came to my class for the first time. While most are shy when they first enter the room, this woman's skepticism held her half-turned toward the door—almost daring me to tell her that she was in the wrong place.

"Yes, it is," I said, "I'm Tari, the teacher."

"Sarah." Her dark eyes watched me closely.

"Welcome, Sarah. Tell me about your cancer."

"Of course," she said. I was happy to see that she brought her whole body to face me.

Addressing the big C right away began the connection I was seeking with Sarah.

"I was diagnosed with breast cancer nearly two years ago," she finally said.

"Are you taking any meds?"

"Yes, tamoxifen. I hate what the drug is doing to my body. I finished chemo a year ago."

"How is it making you feel, the tamoxifen?" I asked.

"Fat, out of shape, and ugly."

"Have you practiced yoga before?"

"I took some yoga classes a number of years ago, but not since I was diagnosed."

"That's okay, new beginnings are great opportunities to find what we really are looking for."

Sarah considered this. . . .

It was a small exchange with a new student, but enough to sense her tension when I asked directly about her cancer. Despite her negative self-image, Sarah was a healthy fifty-four-year-old woman. I invited her to find her mat and join the class.

We began with a restorative backbend, which involves placing the body in a passive but slightly constructed position, using yoga props to gently stretch the spine open in a backward direction. Some women needed more help than others setting up. We all shuffled around making adjustments, getting as comfortable as possible.

I watched the students relax into the pose. Most had their eyes closed, but Sarah's were wide open and locked on me as I worked my way toward the back of the room.

"Yoga," I said, "can seem intimidating when we try it for the first time, or after a long absence from physical activity. Let's start with this supported backbend because it allows everyone an entry point, one that is both familiar and new. Actually, the beginning is you, not the pose. We start with how you are feeling today and where your body is right now—which is here in this space, on your yoga mat."

"Getting here today may have taken some effort: planning, moving a work schedule around, finding a babysitter, or walking out in the cold. But you made it here! Of course, everyone has a different goal—just like every cancer is different, and we are all left with different challenges. Everyone has a different reason."

"What is the same for all of us is a desire to do what we once did, to look the way we once were. That is a good reason to come to yoga, to want to get reacquainted with your body. A natural response in our recovery process is to think we will never be the same again, that our body has somehow let us down."

At this point, I glanced over at Sarah. Now her eyes were closed, but she seemed to be clenching her jaw, her brow slightly furrowed.

"Your body hasn't failed you, but it has changed. Our bodies are constantly changing, with or without cancer. Yoga will help you understand how your body works, what's new about it, and how to feel good about it. Let's use every breath and every pose as an opportunity to turn what may seem impossible into a new normal."

For several minutes I let these words sink in, quietly making tiny adjustments to student props. When I looked back at Sarah again, her jaw was no longer clenched, her brow no longer furrowed. The tension she carried to class was gone.

After class she came up to me with a slight smile and blissful eyes. "It wasn't really an epiphany or anything, but when you said what you did about our bodies always changing, I just felt like I didn't have to judge myself anymore. I had my doubts about this yoga thing, but the class helped me feel that it was okay to be a cancer survivor."

Sarah came to classes over the following weeks. When I greeted her one day, it was clear she already seemed more open, relaxed, and confident.

"Well," she laughed, "I can't let my guard down too much! After class last week, I accidently changed in the men's locker room. I was so blissed-out after class that I didn't notice the looks I was getting from guys standing in their underwear. I realized I was changing in the men's locker room—not the ladies!"

WHY YOGA?

Let's look at the specific benefits of yoga and the supporting research. Given yoga's recent surge of popularity throughout the United States, just about everyone has heard of it. In fact, 20.4 million Americans are enjoying the benefits of yoga every year and another 44.4 percent of Americans plan to do yoga.[1]

We hear about the many ways yoga will make life better, solving all of our physical, mental, and spiritual problems. Claims so broad invite skepticism. Some people, like Sarah, have tested the promises, but remain unsure of the benefits and suspicious of the claims. The valid question Sarah had was: "What could yoga really do for me as a cancer survivor? And why should I believe you?"

My answer to her and to readers is, "Observe the scientific, fact-based principles and benefits of yoga, and test them against personal experience." Before exploring those benefits, let's take a look at the tradition of yoga.

Ask a random person on the street what yoga is, and they might say it's an ancient form of exercise or prayer from India, or that it's a series of forms we make with our body to gain flexibility, or even that it's a class at a gym where people breathe deeply and listen to strange music played on a sitar.

Yoga *is* ancient, and it is widely practiced in India where people use it daily to maintain health and spiritual well-being. It has a rich history with many founders, branches, and varieties practiced around the world. The mysteries of yoga have long been intertwined with the foreign, mystical, and little known beliefs and concepts of Eastern religion and philosophy.

As ancient as yoga is, it is only recently that the West has done research or had an interest in this long tradition of physical and spiritual practice. The y4c methodology introduced here will help ground this ancient practice in Western scientific principles and draw upon empirical research. Actually, my hope is to explain some of those mysteries.

Yoga can be defined as a way to position the body for the purpose of practicing patterned breathing and movement. The goal is to bring balance and alignment to all body parts and systems: muscles, bones, organs, and importantly, the mind. A French geneticist and doctor, Gerard Karsenty, says, "No organ is an island."[2] The interconnection of these organs—the whole body—is where the magic happens! You feel better, stronger, more hopeful, and like Sarah, feel a sense of well-being.

Yoga is a holistic path to wellness focusing on the interconnection of all body systems. Most cancer treatments, like chemotherapy, radiation, or surgeries, are focused on particular points of the body or types of cells. But the treatments can disturb cellular balance or system functions throughout the body, and the effects are not just localized to where a tumor might be or where the treatments are focused. To ignore impact to other body systems does not help those touched by cancer. For example, if Sarah had only focused her physical therapy on where the breast surgeries had been conducted, she would not be addressing the weakness of her bones from chemotherapy and hormone therapy treatments. Yoga helps survivors heal in way that supports wholeness, seeking to strengthen all the systems, both individually and collectively.

Yoga has a spiritual purpose and brings benefits like increased peacefulness for those touched by cancer. These psychological benefits have, in turn, a positive impact on the physical body. For example, reducing anxiety and achieving a greater sense of calmness helps to quiet and strengthen the nervous system. These qualities are tangible, measureable experiences achieved through the practice of yoga. Additionally, being able to move and improve your body provides a strong sense of empowerment and personal control—at a time when most people feel powerless! With y4c yoga it's possible to develop a healthier body and more enjoyable lifestyle than the one before your diagnosis.

Often, the initial cancer does not cause suffering; rather, treatments like surgery or chemotherapy that are designed to control, eliminate, and prevent cancer cell growth can be debilitating. Side effects like scar tissue from a surgery can be uncomfortable, even painful. Most cancer treatments, Western or Eastern, have side effects that can be short term, long term, and even lifelong. Acknowledging them is the first step to recovery. The second step is to learn to manage them rather than surrender.

What are the benefits we seek? Next is an overview of ten benefits of yoga that address common side effects that cancer patients or survivors face on their journey. It is just a sample, but I hope this will awaken your curiosity and understanding. Later in the book specific sample poses, sequences, and practices will be provided to help you apply these benefits and enable you to manage any side effects that you might be facing.

BENEFIT 1:
YOGA DETOXIFIES THE BODY

Detoxification is the metabolic process by which toxins are changed into less toxic substances to be excreted. This is a vital process for everyone, but for cancer survivors, who are dealing with a weakened immune system and undergoing treatments like chemotherapy, radiation, or hormone treatments, this is essential. Whether the goal is to eradicate a flu virus or a potential pathogen, detoxification should be part of every cancer survivor's wellness plan. In chapter 2 we discussed how yoga can apply the science of physics by using the principles of movement, gravity, and resistance to detoxify the body's systems.

These yoga principles utilize and activate the lymphatic system—the body's plumbing and trash-removal system. As mentioned earlier, the lymphatic system has no organ like the heart to circulate its fluids, so it depends on the movement of muscles—especially the heartbeat and the diaphragm muscle—to flush waste or any toxins or potential cancer cells from the body. Yoga increases lymphatic flow by placing the frame of the body in certain postures that move in specific patterns with our muscles. Because muscles need more blood flow when moving than when resting, movement increases the heartbeat. The demand for more blood results in a greater quantity of blood being pumped through the cardiovascular channels located throughout the body. Since the lymph system parallels the cardiovascular system, lymph fluid also flows better when blood flows.

The largest lymph "waste" collector is the thoracic duct located in the body's center. It starts at the bottom of the sternum, below the navel, reaching all the way to the base of the neck. Body movement including diaphragmatic breathing will push and pull the lymph fluid from the arms, legs, and head toward the thoracic duct. From there, lymph fluid is routed through the liver, kidneys, and finally the bladder for discharge. So the aim of yoga practice should be to flush all the lymph canals and nodes, and to aid the flow of lymph fluid in the direction of the thoracic duct.

Gravity also plays a role in detoxification. Inversions of the body such as a modified and supported Shoulderstand are a fundamental part of a strong yoga practice. Inversions utilize movement and body positioning to reverse the effects of gravity on the body, enhancing the process of cardiovascular and lymphatic drainage to your central lymph collector, the thoracic duct. This use of gravity is essential for expelling toxins from the extremities.

Another way yoga detoxifies the body is through compression. I spoke earlier about Iyengar's "squeeze-and-soak" idea—that body twists cleanse internal organs in the same way that a sponge discharges dirty water when squeezed, then reabsorbs fresh water and reexpands. A common utilization of this technique is through abdominal twists that activate internal organs, driving the release of toxins into the lymphatic system.

For all these reasons, detoxification is one of the most important benefits of yoga. In later chapters you will learn poses and sequences to coordinate diaphragmatic breathing with movement to detox the body.

BENEFIT 2:
YOGA STRENGTHENS THE BODY

Cancer treatments like chemotherapy and radiation weaken the body through the process of eliminating cancer as a life-threatening disease. These treatments attack fast-growing cells, but healthy cells, such as bone cells, muscle cells, and the cells of most organs, are also affected. Additionally, during active treatment, people face fatigue that makes normal activity challenging and contributes to further muscle atrophy.

Many methods of building strength exist, from weight lifting to vigorous walking to running. For a cancer patient and survivor, safety is a primary concern; yoga can build strength in a gentle and effective way. For example, yoga uses a person's body weight as resistance, unlike weight lifting. The y4c method eases the body into positions or uses support systems like yoga props, enabling people to build strength over time and without harmful pressure on weakened bones.

Bone Strengthening

Individually, bones are rigid organs; linked together, they form the skeleton, our internal support structure. Bone is living tissue made of calcium and collagens, and it is constantly changing—just like all body parts. New bone cells are always replacing old ones. Bone cells known as osteoblasts build bone and are responsible for maintaining proper bone density. Osteoclasts absorb bone. As we get older, this balance gets disturbed; having thin, weak bones is considered an inevitable part of aging—especially in menopausal women. An overlooked side effect of cancer and its treatment is bone thinning, which happens because the balance of these two cells is disturbed. Remember that chemotherapy is designed to interrupt the activity of cells that multiply. It targets osteoblasts in much the same way it targets cancer cells.[3]

When bones and muscles are not made to work and are not used every day, they do not develop. Worse, deterioration can start quickly, especially as we get older. Research has shown that an excellent solution for weak bones is weight-bearing exercise. In a study conducted at the Hong Kong Polytechnic University in China in 2004, it was shown that regular participation in weight-bearing exercise was beneficial for accruing peak bone mass and optimizing bone structure.[4] Weight-bearing exercises, however, are commonly limited to the kind done with barbells, so the common recommendation to build bones is to lift weights. A recent pilot study that applied yoga practice to sufferers of osteoporosis (decrease in bone mass) and osteopenia (reduction in bone volume) showed that 85 percent of the yoga practitioners gained bone in both the spine and the hip, while nearly every member of the control group either maintained or lost bone mass.[5]

I believe yoga is safer for bone building than many gym routines because it puts weight on the bones in a precise, deliberate way. Following the y4c method, we use our body weight and focus on alignment through simple activities like balancing on one foot. Examples of balancing poses are given in chapter 6 to show how weight-bearing postures can be achieved in a safe and practical way.

Cardiovascular Strength and Fitness

Running is a popular exercise to improve cardiovascular fitness. The goal is to enhance the body's ability to deliver larger amounts of oxygen to working muscles along with burning calories for weight management. Cardiovascular fitness results from the improved efficiency of a lower heart rate and improved oxygenation throughout the body. A 2013 study showed that yoga improved several cardiovascular health markers, like heart rate and respiratory function, at the same level as running.[6] However, running and other high-impact exercises can be risky for cancer patients and survivors due to weakened bones and joints. Running has been proven to contribute to osteoarthritis, an arthritis of the joints that causes swelling and pain.[7] A regular yoga practice can provide the same cardiovascular benefits as running without risk to joints and pain.

Another interesting finding is that heart disease can be reversed, or at least managed, through diet, meditation, and yoga, as reported in *Dr. Dean Ornish's Program for Reversing Heart Disease.* Interestingly, Ornish is now studying whether prostate cancer can be reversed by diet changes and yoga.

Research shows that yoga helps keep a heart healthy and strong. Unlike the gentle and restorative yoga that is usually recommended for cancer survivors, y4c yoga focuses on patterned movement, ranging from slow and gentle to active, which sometimes may appear similar to cardiovascular exercise. Heart rate and breathing increase, and people sweat! One example is modified Sun Salutations, a sequence of yoga poses designed to move the spine, arms, and legs in precise directions combined with deep breathing. The body moves, the heart beats, blood flows, and the breath deepens—all combining to build a strong heart muscle.

BENEFIT 3: YOGA INCREASES RANGE OF MOTION AND FLEXIBILITY

As a yoga teacher, I hear one thing all the time: "I can't do yoga because I'm not flexible!" People say this before they're diagnosed with cancer or even if they are not given a cancer diagnosis. A flexible body is a useful body because we can do more with it, moving bones freely and without pain. We want to be able to reach for that shoebox on the top shelf, or bend over to tie our shoes.

Cancer treatments, however, can reduce flexibility because surgeries and radiation create scar tissue around muscles and joints. The scarring can make the body stiff and painful to move. Other treatments like chemotherapy and hormone therapy create joint stiffness, which decrease the body's ability to bend, limiting the ability of muscles and bones to work together efficiently. All of these problems make life's daily and necessary functions difficult, such as being able to walk the dog or move a chair. In fact, we consider ourselves recovered from cancer when we have resumed normal activities.

A yoga practice will improve flexibility, making movement easier. Like a parked car that will not move if it sits on its wheels for eight months, we must keep the joints moving and the muscles stretching or else they "rust." (Actually, if we do not use muscles, they deteriorate more rapidly than we imagine.) What we learn is how to become more flexible by changing habits that prevent flexibility as well as learning how to protect ourselves as we reach our goals. This approach is designed to increase flexibility and to regain and maintain mobility in daily life.

The y4c method looks at body movement in a logical, patterned way. Movements are slow, gentle, and supported, with careful attention placed on the position of the bones relative to the muscles. Increasing range of motion happens by alternating the extension and flexion of muscles, combined with patterned movement. This method helps you explore and regain your range of motion, and improve strength and flexibility in general. It also includes passive, restorative poses that use gravity to increase flexibility. These well-supported poses also soothe muscles. The purpose is for you to be able to go about your daily life activities with less pain and more confidence.

BENEFIT 4:
YOGA KEEPS THE SPINE STRONG

Having correct posture not only makes you look younger, but it keeps you healthier. Posture is the position in which we stack the bones of the spine (vertebrae) and use muscles to keep them in place. When we properly align the body, the spine takes on a beautiful, natural S curve. When we let the body slump, we change the spine's shape and restrict body systems like digestion, causing us to look and feel unhealthy. Bad posture limits and crowds the space necessary for lungs, stomach, intestines, and even the heart to function. We need oxygen to feed our cells, and we need our gastrointestinal system to be unrestricted so it can remove potential carcinogens from foods we have consumed. With good posture, adequate space exists for all the organs to work together. And in this way, good posture aids detoxification.

Yoga teaches us to align the bones of our spine to create good posture in every pose and movement. We also learn to use the breath to make the spine and the rest of the musculoskeletal system strong. The first step, however, is to take an honest look at your posture, like I did. This will help you determine the state of your S curve.*

This book encourages deliberate exploration of the body's skeletal structure to create proper alignment and good posture. We will refine the techniques of movement through five natural and healthy directions in which to move the whole spine and keep it strong. They are: lengthening upward and downward, bending forward, bending backward, bending sideways, and twisting around the spinal column.

A recent Norwegian study confirms the benefits of yoga on vertebral fractures and osteoporosis. But the research warns that a practice that is too aggressive or forceful could be harmful, leading to compression of the spine.[8] This is why y4c methodology focuses on supported poses and deliberate alignment to ensure that the spine is not put under too much stress. For example, we encourage a supported forward bend with blocks in order to protect lower vertebrae while enabling a student to gain the benefits of a forward bend. (Review extension, flexion, and twisting as part of the science behind yoga in chapter 2, pages 48–49.)

Finally, developing back strength for correct posture is essential for breast cancer survivors after axillary node surgeries (which I had) or breast reconstruction surgery (which I passed up). These procedures leave women (and some men) with significant scar tissue, reducing strength on both sides of the torso. Women who have undergone reconstructive surgery can face months of rehabilitation, pain, and restricted movement. After my surgeries, my arm movement was restricted and I regained range of motion and strength with my yoga practice. Because breast cancer is the most newly diagnosed form of cancer that affects 29 percent of women with cancer,[9] y4c methodology emphasizes improving flexibility, regaining range of motion, and reducing scar tissue for the upper body. Without careful focus on and consistent maintenance of abdominal and back muscles, the spine can become compromised, thus impacting other functions such as balance, breathing capacity, circulation of blood and lymph fluid, and proper digestion.

---

*Some helpful references on posture and back care are *Back Care Basics* by Mary Pullig Schatz, M.D. (Berkeley, CA: Rodmell Press, 1992), *Anatomy of Hatha Yoga* by H. David Coulter (Marlboro, VT: Body and Breath, 2010), and *Cure Back Pain with Yoga* by Loren Fishman, M.D., and Carol Ardman (New York: W. W. Norton & Co., 2005).

BENEFIT 5: YOGA
STRENGTHENS THE IMMUNE SYSTEM

Many people make the claim that if you practice yoga, you will strengthen the immune system. Often these claims are not substantiated by knowledge of what the immune system is and how it works. Let's explore the ways in which cancer and treatments for cancer impair the immune system and how yoga practice bolsters it.

As discussed earlier, the immune system is not a single, tangible part of the body like the lungs, heart, brain, or stomach. In one sense, the immune system includes all of the body's parts and systems, being the interaction and union of all these systems. The goal of strengthening the immune system is to keep all the systems working together, like working families in a large, healthy village. In chapter 2, we said the failure of any one system threatens the health of the whole community—for example, if our bones are compromised from a break or osteoporosis (a side effect of chemotherapy) we will not be able produce new nourishing blood supply to feed our reproducing cells. Additionally, we learned how the immune system is constantly on the lookout for a new or returning cancer cell.

Chemotherapy and other cancer treatments can compromise the immune system's efficiency because they disrupt the development and balance of all cells, therefore stressing the body's systems and increasing the risk of infection or other diseases. Specifically, treatments reduce white cells in the blood that are needed to form leukocytes, a natural immune protection. This is why it is so critical for active cancer patients to keep on "immune system alert." Because yoga's goal is to strengthen all body systems, the end product is an improved immune system.

On a molecular level, we find further support that yoga boosts the immune system. Recent research has found that yoga causes an improvement in gene expression within lymphocytes, which are our cancer-fighting cells, often referred to as immune cells, that are being produced in our body all the time.[10] Gene expression "is the process by which information from a gene is used to make a functional gene product,"[11] which in this case is to aid lymphocyte production. In this science-based way yoga boosts our natural defense against cancer. Every y4c yoga movement, position, or patterned breathing technique has one goal: to strengthen the immune system!

BENEFIT 6:
YOGA HELPS MANAGE WEIGHT GAIN

When people think of cancer patients, they imagine skinny, fragile bodies. And yes, this is often the case during active treatment, prolonged treatment, or late stages of cancer. But for many people, weight gain is a common side effect of cancer treatment. Weight gain has significant impact on both physical and psychological aspects of a survivor's life. However, an additional great concern of weight gain is possible recurrence.

Obesity is a key indicator of both cancer incidence and recurrence. The American Cancer Society recommends that obese individuals increase the standard weekly exercise from 150 minutes to 300 minutes per week to reduce the chances of cancer or recurrence.[12] Thus managing one's weight should be a focus of any cancer patient or survivor (and everyone in general).

Yoga provides a safe, gentle way to manage weight. Research on the impact of yoga on weight gain is still in early stages. One study showed that yoga had a more positive impact on obesity (and depression) than aerobic exercise.[13]

But not all yoga is the same. And I would not argue that all styles will help you manage weight gain. Often, yoga for cancer survivors is focused on gentle or restorative yoga methods, which are necessary and beneficial approaches. But these do not provide an *active* yoga practice. Many yoga teachers are afraid to make cancer patients and survivors move and be active in class.

It is a mistake to coddle survivors, treating them as sick. I remember this from my own days of attending a yoga class, with my bald head and the teacher encouraging me to lie in restorative poses and not participate in the active yoga class. I felt isolated, ashamed, and annoyed. Worse, if I had listened to my teacher, I would not have benefited fully from the active yoga practice. Therefore, including an active practice is the foundation of y4c methodology.

Yoga for cancer survivors can be active, therefore calorie burning; and it can be safe, physically accessible, welcoming, and inclusive. Yoga can help cancer survivors manage weight gain, which improves self-esteem and the ability to function normally, and ultimately reduces the risk of recurrence. Chapter 8 (pages 255–58) includes poses to help you do this.

BENEFIT 7: YOGA HELPS MANAGE PAIN

Dorothy is a tall, attractive Polish woman who is fifty-four years old. She had a double mastectomy when she was fifty-two, which was then followed by eight months of chemotherapy and radiation treatments. She tests positive for BRAC 1, the breast cancer gene. Her mother died of breast cancer at age forty-seven. Dorothy expressed concern to me before a recent yoga class about a new pain she was experiencing in her shoulder blades. As if whispering a secret, she asked me if it could be cancer. I was not surprised by her question, but asked her if she felt any pain when two years earlier she detected her breast cancer. "No," she said, "Only a lump. . . . "

It is not easy to listen to the body. We get so many aches and pains before, during, and after cancer. Most are not caused by cancer, but that is the fear. As survivors we are hyper-alert to new body sensations and naturally, we worry. The nervous system is a tricky alarm system sending signals that are sometimes confusing, false, or, as was the case with Dorothy, misunderstood.

Until advanced stages, most cancers do not cause pain. Rather, the treatments and their side effects can cause pain, not the cancer itself. Acknowledging this fact and then applying curiosity mixed with practical information helps us manage our pain as well as our fears. In my conversations with Dorothy later on, she realized that the pain she was feeling, although real, was not due to cancer. Rather, it was a strained back muscle! During class, we did many poses and patterned movements that gave her relief and insights into how she was using her shoulder and arm.

But a yoga practice can reduce pain. Studies have concluded that yoga can help reduce pain for both non-cancer and cancer populations.[14] The y4c methodology modifies traditional yoga poses so that you can practice with less pain. You will learn tips to help you manage body sensations and to modify poses according to *your* body's needs and the changing circumstances of your recovery.

BENEFIT 8:
YOGA HELPS MANAGE FEAR AND ANXIETY

Fear is one of the most common and overwhelming reactions to those three little words, "You have cancer." For most of us, if not all of us, it puts us into a tailspin of fear of pain, the impact on family, loss of income, and ultimately, death. As a cancer survivor adjusts to a life-threatening disease, an additional alarm system emerges: uncertainty. From that point on, every tweak, pain, or twitch, even old familiar ones, creates anxiety. Anxiety about what is and is not cancer becomes a new threat and constant companion. This undercurrent of anxiety and fear impact mood, causes depression, and affects quality and length of sleep. These then impact our body's natural systems to heal and restore, further weakening a survivor's physical and psychological status. It's a nasty downward spiral.

Yoga is well known for its powers of relaxation. Many are unaware of the physical benefits, though they are easily understood and recognized in popular and modern culture. I want to provide some fact-based reasons for why yoga can help reduce anxiety and fear to essentially calm the nervous system.

The nervous system is a complex network of trillions of cells and countless communication pathways throughout the body. Information is delivered to the brain in the form of sensations through sight, hearing, tasting, smelling, touching, and feeling. And the body responds to these sensations, or signals, with pleasure or discomfort and pain. Both responses are interpretations made by the brain to protect us from harm, maximize health, and enhance well-being. If we were in freezing weather and didn't have a nervous system, we wouldn't know how cold we were and wouldn't protect ourselves with winter clothing, risking serious conditions like hypothermia. Without the nervous system, we would not know what is happening in the body, and it would be impossible to take care of ourselves. So an anxious nervous system not only impacts the way we emotionally feel but how our body functions and the power of our immune system.

Research about yoga's positive impact on the nervous system, especially in reducing anxiety and fear, is plentiful. In 2013 a study conducted by the University of Calgary showed that practicing yoga led to improvements in mood, stress factors, and health-related quality of life (HRQL).[15] Participants saw an improvement within the seven-week trial and then in three- and six-month follow-ups. Another study suggests that yoga can be more effective on mood than walking, which is a common recommendation for cancer patients and survivors. Yoga participants reported greater improvement in mood and a reduction in anxiety levels over the control group that only walked.[16]

Anxiety causes sleep disruption. It's estimated that between 30 percent and 90 percent of cancer survivors have problems sleeping. A study published in the *Journal of Clinical Oncology* in 2013 reported that 90 percent of cancer survivors who participated in a yoga program saw improvement in their sleep; they had better sleep quality, less daytime sleepiness, better quality of life, and reduced use of medicines.[17]

Some psychological principles that help us are the relaxation response, the power of positive expectations, and pranayama, breath control using the practice of various breathing techniques. The latter is a key technique for inducing relaxation in the body. This is the science behind yoga that invites you to enjoy safe and relaxing positions, respect your body, settle the monkey mind, work past the normal distractions of daily life, better manage fears and anxiety, and help you make time for healing.

Survivor Story

Like two race cars colliding, my life prior to my endometrial cancer diagnosis and my life post radical hysterectomy explosively barreled into one another, engulfing me in flames. Emotionally decimated by this crash, I tried to make sense of an equation that failed to add up. How could I go back to being who I was before this diagnosis and who had I become as a result?

It was my sophomore year of college. Typically a good student, I normally found solace in my reading and writing. Now I struggled to read or write at all. I felt alienated from my peer group and suffered from extreme anxiety while trying to focus on my studies. Even though I tried to maintain a positive attitude, feeling grateful that the doctors caught my cancer early and my surgery successfully eliminated the malignant growth, my confidence collapsed like a sand castle built too close to the incoming tide.

I felt fragmented, unable to communicate what I was going through. I wanted my energy, focus, concentration, and sense of self back. I took a leave of absence from my classes to take care of my health and rebuild my stamina. During my time off, I began reading books on yoga and practicing asana by myself at night before bed. Soon after, I found my body on a rented, well-worn, black sticky mat in a tiny yoga studio for the very first time. Thereafter, my yoga practice gradually became a part of my daily life, a non-negotiable. It rescued the girl set ablaze in the aftermath of cancer. With a growing practice in place, I returned to college and successfully completed my studies.

Slowly, with my practice, I released the trauma of surgical menopause in my teenage years. I developed a connection with my breath that granted me access to a deeper experience of both my body and my spirit, previously inaccessible. Learning how to move my body in alignment with my breath liberated me from the restriction of incomplete, shallow inhalations, and an inability to witness my body in motion. I learned how to live in motion and flow with change. My yoga asana practice midwifed my relationship with my body after cancer. Releasing constrictions and gaining expansion helped me to assimilate who I was becoming in the aftermath of cancer. I met the new me on my mat, and it's been a relationship of true love ever since.

BENEFIT 9:
YOGA ENHANCES BODY IMAGE

People have images from news media and film of people practicing yoga. Perhaps we picture limber, lean, and youthful bodies in tights and tank tops sitting cross-legged or bent completely backward like a human Gateway Arch in St. Louis. Celebrities and famous athletes do it. Everybody under thirty seems to be doing it. These young people might think they look like a model on the cover of *Yoga Journal,* and the serene look on their faces suggests that they're not just in good physical shape, but their minds are in good shape too.

I believe yoga makes us feel good from the inside out. Yoga does not just help the body get strong, flexible, and detoxified. It helps our perception of the body and improves self-esteem. Cancer survivors, especially those who have survived breast cancer, have the same desire as everyone else: to look good! And yoga *is* for ordinary bodies. However, when baldness is not a fashion statement and makes us look sick, or when we feel weak, have gained twenty pounds from medical treatments, or have lost body parts, feeling good about how we look seems out of reach. Encouraging survivors to find a way to feel good about their appearance may sound unrealistic.

Rather than feel good, some survivors feel shame or embarrassment by their disfigurement. They say their body has betrayed them, as if blaming it helps explain a terrifying, mysterious disease. Survivors might also blame—falsely—their will, instead of their body, and think that they did not eat enough organic food, take enough vitamins and supplements, or use enough alternative therapies. Feelings of failure are not helpful and only add stress to life.

Here is what I have learned. Not only has the body not betrayed us, but by thinking this way we risk just such a betrayal. Research on stress and emotion suggests how a negative attitude toward oneself causes stress hormones to rise, thus increasing the risk for cancer.[18] Even though research progress is being made, we know less than we should about what causes cancer. Almost always, it is not possible to identify the exact causes for an individual cancer. Rather, the best we can do is to manage risk. What we do know, though, is that having positive thoughts cannot hurt us.[19]

So, a y4c yoga practice seeks to free the mind of negative thoughts and feelings about our bodies. Instead of looking into the mirror and making poor comparisons to magazine cover models, yoga teaches us how to turn the mirror around to find what is hidden on the inside. When we do something every day, even if it is a simple stretch, breathing exercise, or correcting our posture while walking down the street, we develop a healthier, more positive image of our-selves. This is how yoga starts to work and over time, will enhance your body image. By having a daily yoga practice, either alone or with others, survivors see what is good on the inside. A virtuous cycle of positive benefits results.

BENEFIT 10: YOGA ENHANCES EMPOWERMENT AND WELL-BEING

Many have heard of post-traumatic stress disorder (PTSD), a condition experi-enced by some soldiers returning from war, or by people suffering from a life-threatening accident. Cancer patients and survivors experience similar stress. We feel bombarded by frightening information, subjected to invasive proce-dures, and must endure cold clinics and blank stares.

Not everyone though manages stress with the same success, and a 2009 study by Costanzo, Ryff, and Singer developed and tested a concept that mea-sures how we respond to post-traumatic stress growth, the positive flip side to suffering with stress.[20] The researchers categorized the elements of surviving stressful events in three ways: survival with impairment, survival with resil-ience, and survival by thriving. Surviving with impairment, a survivor may blame her trauma on everything wrong with life. Surviving with resilience means she may recover from the trauma and live a serviceable life. Surviving by thriving, though, occurs when people make the traumatic event a pivotal point in life, changing their situation by making lemonade out lemons—ulti-mately thriving after cancer, for instance. The thriving survivor enjoys her blissful moments, which can lead to further change and the ability to find positive ways to manage stress.

About managing stress and cancer, Suzanne Danhauer of Wake Forest School of Medicine says, "Given the high levels of stress and distress that cancer patients experience, the opportunity to feel more peaceful and calm is a sig-nificant benefit."[21] She goes on to describe results of random trials studying the effects of yoga on emotions. Her research, conducted in 2009, found an increase of positive emotions such as calmness and a sense of purpose in over 50 percent of her subjects.

So, a growing body of research shows that yoga provides emotional ben-efits. Whether we use yoga to lose weight gained by taking medication, to detox our body following chemotherapy, or to regain the use of our arms, practicing yoga helps us feel better. As these benefits become more apparent, we experience increased well-being and, more importantly, feel more empowered than before.

A positive spiral toward health results; as we continue to feel better, we make even better decisions about how to bring balance and ease to our lives.

Often, survivors with a yoga practice are surprised to find self-healing and empowerment in addition to their newfound well-being. Yoga empowers us to define life on our own terms. A solid practice can help reduce drug dependency or leave us feeling like we had a great massage. Ultimately, yoga helps us create a sense of balance between body and mind, the physical and the spiritual.

A final point: The first obstacle to exploring the great promises of a yoga practice is accepting that things are never going to be the same—and that is okay. Learning how to practice self-compassion is the most important benefit of all, what I call the *bliss* benefit.

MOVING FORWARD
WITH YOUR YOGA PRACTICE

I believe that yoga helps us recover and learn to manage life, which will always have surprises. The promise of the benefits described in this chapter sound nice, and they may even sound similar to promises made by others who tout yoga as exercise. Ultimately, a y4c yoga practice can lead to benefits that you can adapt to your needs. The following chapters provide you with all of the tools necessary to enjoy these benefits—and many more—as you become a thriving survivor.

To end this chapter, we return to Sarah's story. She continued to come to class over the next several months. During that time she told me that getting breast cancer had made her feel like she had lost the life that she once enjoyed. Working through her condition had been a matter of struggling to reclaim what that life had been, doing so in any way she could. As she returned to class each week, she found a way to reverse her recent weight gain, restore range of motion, and gain self-confidence. Just as important, she realized that class was an opportunity to pay attention to herself in a way that she had not ever done before. Through yoga, Sarah found a way to connect to her body, a sense of community, and a feeling of bliss. "Yoga doesn't really change you," Sarah said to me one day. "It helps you to discover who you really are."

PART 2

How to Build Your Own Yoga Practice

If cancer is life's reset button,
then yoga is the jump start.

TARI PRINSTER

The next four chapters are the heart of my book. It is time to get moving! You will read about specific poses that are beneficial for survivors and other poses that should be avoided or used only with caution. Our focus is building your personal yoga practice that you can apply at home or in a class. As I did in Part 1, I will draw upon personal examples from my own practice, from my teaching with survivors and at teacher trainings all around the country, and from my own cancer path.

In the beginning of this section, I will present five principles—the y4c theory—and seven building blocks—the elements—of creating the best healing practice. Together they are the foundation upon which anyone can formulate a yoga practice and modify yoga to meet their needs. This foundation developed over time as my own yoga practice evolved, while observing thousands of cancer survivors and helping each cultivate an appropriate yoga practice.

Now I want to help you begin a personal practice to reduce stress, detox your body, improve your sense of balance, build strong bones and muscles, and allow you to begin to take control of your recovery. Most important of all, we will use yoga poses and sequences of poses to strengthen the immune system to improve quality of life and help you manage cancer. I want you to feel whole again—and in control!

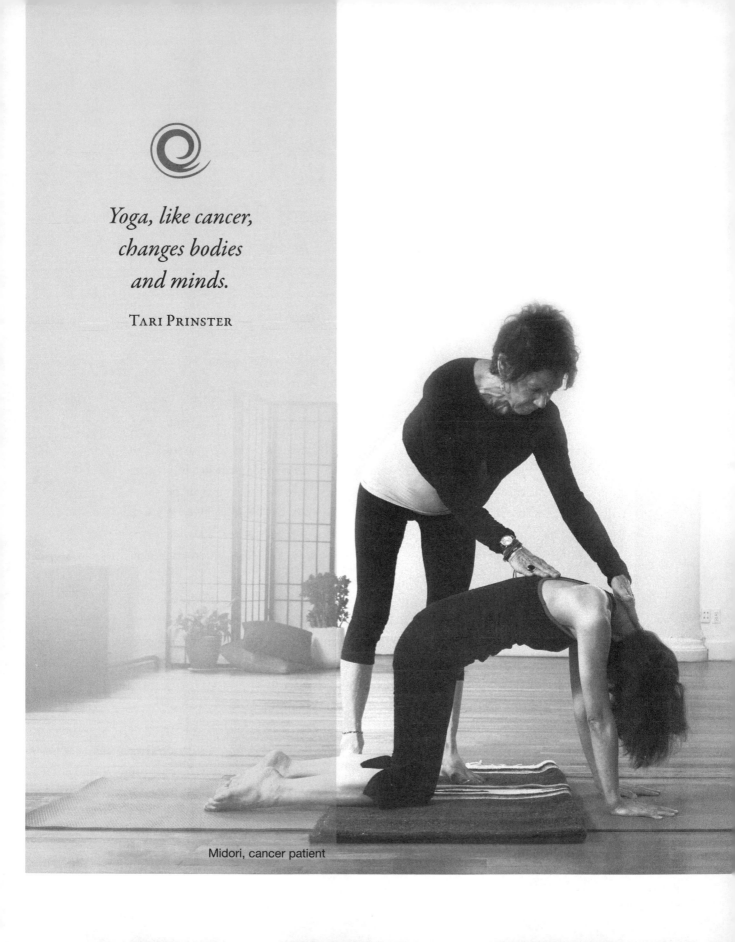

Yoga, like cancer, changes bodies and minds.

TARI PRINSTER

Midori, cancer patient

4

The y4c (yoga4cancer) Methodology

FIVE PRINCIPLES OF Y4C METHODOLOGY

The methodology of y4c is based on five principles that I describe below. In addition to giving guidance, these principles have a surprising connection to the Hindu concept of the *koshas*. *Kosha* in Sanskrit, an ancient language that originated in India, means "envelope or sheath" and refers to the energetic layers of the body. In Vedantic philosophy of Hinduism, these sheaths protect and embody our physical and psychological experiences throughout life. The five koshas are containers of knowledge that inform the five principles.

Principle 1:
Using the Breath to Heal—Pranamaya Kosha

Pranamaya kosha is the energy layer. In Sanskrit *prana* translates to breath. According to yoga traditions, prana metaphorically means the vital life-force that flows through, enlivens, and maintains all our physical systems. Everyone has a first breath. They also have a last. Breathing fills every second of our lives. Yet most of us take breathing for granted. We think we do not need lessons in how to breathe. But to make breathing a healing activity and to improve its quality, there is much to learn. When explored in the context of cancer survival, breathing is much more than life sustaining. Breathing with awareness—mindful breathing—will be one of your most vital tools in cancer recovery.

Mindful breathing can be used to reduce the anxiety and stress that come with cancer and its treatments. It is a way to feel safe and hopeful rather than challenged. Personally, I learned mindful breathing to reduce the fear I felt when getting prepped for chemotherapy. The antihistamine administered before the chemo made me anxious, but my healing breathing calmed my nerves and allowed me to set aside my fears without the use of drugs. If you incorporate a conscious breathing routine into your practice, it may also improve your body's reaction to treatments, reducing the potential for harmful side effects.

Chapter 2 helped you understand how the breath functions mechanically in the body, making it a tool for healing and for staying healthy. Mindful breathing will aid in cultivating a cancer *unfriendly* environment in the body, which is your best tool to prevent a recurrence—the ultimate goal of every survivor.

Principle 2:
The Moving Body—Annamaya Kosha

The *annamaya kosha* is the physical body. In the second principle of y4c yoga, this is where we start movement of the physical body in the practice of yoga. Just as our breath gives us energy and life from outside the body, movement creates an energy level starting inside the body and keeps us alive. After treatments, patients are told to go home and take it easy. I know I was. Caretakers and family members coddle the patient into a sedentary attitude without recognizing that the body has evolved to move as well as rest. Our job as survivors is simple: *keep the immune system healthy!* Movement is one essential, natural way to do that and to keep the body unfriendly to cancer.

As I mentioned earlier, our bodies were designed to move and when we do so in a healthy way, we massage organs and detox body systems like the heart, lungs, and lymph nodes. Lack of movement endangers both the body and the mind. We will show you how specific movement will lead to a healthy body. Research data, we have seen, is conclusive that exercise can modify human emotions, creating feelings of well-being. So, a strong body and a positive mind together become the healing power of the second principle.

Cancer survivors need to be aware of specific movement in response to treatments, surgeries, and other changes in the body that have taken place. The yoga poses outlined here have been tailored to provide a structure for overcoming the many obstacles associated with these changes and side effects, both short and long term.

Chapter 5 will give you a basic vocabulary of yoga poses that are later used to create patterned movement and introduce you to the best poses. I give simple, straightforward instructions for each pose to ensure that you feel confident moving your body in these new ways and to overcome any fears and misconceptions about movement you may have now, or have had in the past. And in chapter 6, you will learn how to use the poses to create a yoga practice specific to your needs.

Principle 3:
Body Mind Wisdom—Manomaya Kosha

Mana means mind. *Manomaya kosha* is the energetic layer of the body where we absorb, process, and interpret input from the physical body. Through our five senses we experience everything we know. The mind is stimulated by a continuous stream of sensations all day and night. It fluctuates among these many sensations, trying to make sense of them. Is it raining? Am I hungry? What is that tingle in my left toe? As a cancer survivor adjusts to the news of a life-threatening disease, a new alarm system emerges in relation to sensations, especially pain. Every type of pain that the survivor has—even old and familiar ones—becomes a new fear of having cancer. Uncertainty becomes a new companion.

The third principle recognizes that cancer leads to emotional side effects, not just physical ones. Yoga will teach you to observe sensations in your body, how to resist being distracted by them, and how to monitor them.

The word *mindful* comes up frequently in my book and in the yoga community, where it can have different meanings.* I use it to mean that the mind is full . . . full of something, full of thoughts and ideas. That is all it can contain— thoughts. Because we know the world through the body, the third principle draws attention or awareness to the ability of the body to control the mind. We

---

*Different definitions of mindfulness exist, as well as growing empirical support for its benefits in healing and education. Mindfulness in the Buddhist tradition has been written about for hundreds of years. For an introduction, read Thich Nhat Hanh's *The Miracle of Mindfulness: An Introduction to the Practice of Meditation*. Lately, mindfulness has become a popular topic for Western clinical researchers like Jon Kabat-Zinn and social psychologists like Ellen Langer who refer to a flexible way of thinking about the world without preconditions.

need to cultivate a mind full of *properly placed* thoughts. We can place thoughts in our mind and we can take thoughts out of our mind. For example, a thought that causes anxiety, such as fear of a cancer recurrence, could be replaced by a thought of well-being by taking five slow, calming breaths every time that thought places itself in your mind. And we need to have a mind determined to use that information to heal. Yoga will help you train your mind to be mindful about everything you do and think.

Having questions about the how and why of anything is the best use of the mind. In relation to yoga and cancer, questions like, "Why is yoga beneficial to cancer survivors?" and "How can yoga heal or make our bodies more resistant to cancer?" are helpful. This is how we want the mind to work rather than having fear of developing a new cancer.

The answers are found in learning how to listen and observe the body. In yoga, we sometimes do things that seem unfamiliar, maybe slightly uncomfortable. Listening to your body in those situations—at the same time, knowing why you are doing so—will make the experience more empowering, meaningful, and positive. This is how yoga trains the mind. If you are able to quiet your mind and hear your body speak, then a healing process unfolds that is empowering and life preserving. The mind will give witness to the information your body gathers. Together, they will be wise and potentially healing.

Principle 4:
Connecting Wisdom—Vijnanamaya Kosha

Vijnana means knowing and takes consciousness to a higher level. It is here that the reactive, reflective mind guides and integrates our experience into the world around us. The sheath that shelters our vulnerabilities is the fourth principle. Being with others takes us out of that emotional sheath. What material would you use to make a protective sheath around your emotions? If that were possible, it would need to be strong, sensitive, supportive, patient, and wise. The container for all the possible feelings that arise after a cancer diagnosis must also be flexible and stable. We feel so many emotions, each requiring special consideration.

Cancer can be a lonely, long path. You feel, look, and think of yourself as different. Family and friends treat you that way. Before diagnosis, you may not have known others who have been on the cancer path. But taking this trip alone is unnecessary. This principle of y4c is about learning ways to connect with other people in order to feel part of a community.

There is a benefit to interacting with other survivors living with and overcoming similar challenges. Connecting with others helps us understand ourselves, and helps us heal both emotionally and physically. Embarrassed by disfigurement, hair loss, weight gain, or weight loss; feeling fatigued, scared, and alone—this is a small sampling of the emotions we share as cancer survivors.* Support groups are ways of creating community that can enhance quality of life for survivors, including reducing pain and helping to create a positive mood.[1] Community protects and allows us to understand our emotions. Learning with, and from, others makes us stronger.

Principle 5:
Self-Compassion and Bliss—Anandamaya Kosha

Ananda means bliss. *Anandamaya kosha* is considered the emotional energy level of unbounded peacefulness and contentment. The fifth principle of y4c methodology is the act of being kind to yourself—self-compassion. We'll discuss how to practice self-compassion to experience contentment and bliss. Everyone comes to yoga seeking something. I believe survivors come to yoga seeking comfort and hope as well as strength and healing. Frequently, they leave feeling good and empowered. Yoga promises and usually delivers, in my experience. It also suggests something more is possible beyond the sensory experience. There are those who call that something enlightenment or happiness. In my teaching, I call it *bliss*, or the feeling of contentment. It gives hope because it begins with the gesture of being loving toward yourself.

The world is full of suffering. And the world puts obstacles in our paths. It is continuously jabbing us with expectations and illuminating all the ways in which we need to improve, have more, look better, and be worried about the future. All of these are obstacles to feeling happy and content. Cancer only adds more obstacles.

Whatever label we use—enlightenment, bliss, or happiness—having comfort and hope is essential to being well and content with the life we have. Wellness is health. That is the first physical motivation to come to yoga. Perhaps the subtle, hidden gem of yoga is contentment.

What is contentment? The word *contain* in Old English means "everything inside a container." It is the contents of you! Cultivating contentment is being aware of yourself, being comfortable inside the space that is you. With yoga we learn how to be comfortable in that space. We learn to accept and appreciate the contents of ourselves and what we find at any given moment.

*Depression may make the effects of cancer worse, according to David Spiegel. For more information, go to http://med.stanford.edu/ism/2009/august/depression.html.

Finding enlightenment, bliss, and happiness starts with the most personal and purest gift to the most important person, you. It is not self-centeredness to be kind to yourself; it is the foundation of life and the beginning of love. It is the first step to finding hope.

Yoga also helps you learn how to respond to the thoughts, feelings, and expectations of your senses that feed your mind, in a way that allows you to not respond to distracting thoughts. Learning to be nonresponsive to the emotions of the moment offers you a moment of relief, or a second of "bliss." That is what others may refer to as enlightenment. The first step is learning to see what is on the inside, the beauty and life within the body. The second step is learning to appreciate all that we are, all that we really have, and still have.

Enlightenment comes to a survivor when she recognizes that things are never going to be the same, but to acknowledge that this is okay. When that happens, a precious opening is made, one that allows the rest of the world to see our contentment. That is the light, the bliss, the glow. Chapter 5 expands on these general principles and gives you concrete steps for building your own yoga practice.

Survivor Story

I like to have things planned. Call it being prepared, call it being a control freak, I've always liked being ready rather than surprised. Then all of a sudden, out of nowhere, I was diagnosed with lung cancer at age thirty-nine. Surprise!

Even more troubling, the cancer had an extra year-and-a-half head start because my busy doctor never told me that my CT scan revealed a suspicious node in my lung. After noticing a strange pain in my chest following a yoga headstand, I asked for a physical copy of the eighteen-month-old CT scan report and discovered what the doctor never read or told me. The CT scan report focused on a suspicious nodule with many characteristics that are consistent with cancer and called for further testing. With a disease like cancer, catching and treating the disease early can be a matter of life and death. When questioned, the doctor admitted that somehow my case had "slipped through the cracks."

I had always had incredible faith in doctors and the medical system as a whole until I discovered this hole in the system. Now the news ripped a hole through my life.

I was the mother of a daughter at a new school, the wife of a husband starting up a new business, and I was in the middle of training for a new career as a yoga instructor. My whole world was so full of exciting change when the news of cancer changed my whole worldview. I had a potentially life-threatening, time-sensitive medical condition that was given an unnecessary eighteen-month opportunity to take hold in my lung and spread throughout my body.

From the time I finally received my scan results in the mail to the time I had my lung surgery to remove the nodule, I was devastated, furious, and petrified. I had to watch my daughter knowing that I may be dying. I smiled through my daughter's fifth birthday party not knowing if I would be at her sixth. I hoped my husband would be strong enough if he had to raise her without me. It was hard to think straight and stay off the computer researching what my possible fate might be.

A second CT scan found the nodule had grown over the last eighteen months—not a good sign. Cancer grows. A PET scan "lit up," also pointing toward malignancy. I was referred to a highly recommended thoracic surgeon in Los Angeles. He performed video-assisted thoracoscopic surgery (VATS) to remove the nodule soon after.

On July 21, 2011, one-third of my left upper lung was removed along with four lymph nodes. Lab tests eventually led to a diagnosis of stage 1 mucinous adenocarcinoma with bronchioloalveolar carcinoma (BAC) features. BAC is a unique subtype of lung cancer that seems to strike a higher demographic of young women than other forms of lung cancer.

Recovering from surgery was more difficult than I expected. I had terrible side effects from the pain medicines and ended up convulsing in my hospital bed. I could not stand on my legs or lift my left arm. I had never had surgery before and now I had a tube sticking out of my chest cavity draining fluids for days.

Through all the emotional and physical upheaval, I was fortunate to have an amazing support system. My husband never left my side and was truly my advocate and rock in a very confusing, frightening time. The yoga school where I was doing my teacher training was very flexible and I was able to simply postpone my graduation. My daughter was in summer camp and we had support from her old school in Los Angeles as well as her summer camp in Las Vegas. We were lucky to have the love and support of our families and friends to help us through.

After surgery I was unable to drive a car or lift anything close to heavy; being a stay-at-home mom made that very difficult. I had my best friend,

Lane, come out from Minneapolis to stay with us for a week to help out. Friends sent us food, picked up our mail, and sent encouraging words. I was incredibly frustrated and upset with the limitations of my physical body and the pain that I was in. It took a full eight weeks to recover, but the one thing that helped me the most with my focus, my hopes, and my healing process was yoga.

From my yoga practice over the years I knew how yoga could help me, but I was too much of a mess to focus and help myself. I needed someone to guide me. I was lucky to find a healing yoga class taught by an amazing teacher named Helen. She has volunteered twice a week for seven years and her classes are packed. I was afraid and angry as I walked through her doors, and as she turned down the lights and rang her meditation bell, the tears finally began to flow. Her warm, nurturing manner and genuine concern for me was overwhelming, and I finally felt like I belonged somewhere in my newly sick body. After class, a young woman named Alice came up to me and introduced herself, and we have become very close friends ever since. Her twenty-year journey with cancer has been incredibly tough, but she finds solace in the healing yoga classes as well. She has been a true inspiration to me.

Yoga teaches us that we are exactly where we are supposed to be: an impossible idea to believe in when you are a cancer survivor; however, a beautiful idea to hold onto when the rest of the world wants you to "get well soon!" Recovery from cancer can take a long time, and I don't feel like we actually "recover" as much as we learn ways to cope. Yoga teaches us to listen to our bodies and they will eventually heal in their own time.

When I went to yoga after my surgery, for the first time I could not take a full breath due to the loss of lung capacity, and I was in too much pain to lie on my back. I couldn't lift my left arm and I couldn't wear a bra or stop crying. Nobody treated me like I was different. I looked forward to going to that class every Tuesday and Thursday because I could breathe, I could relax, I could cry, and I could nurture my body, and slowly my body began to return to normal.

It has been six months since my diagnosis, and not only have I returned to my regular yoga classes, but I have become certified in teaching yoga to cancer survivors as well as getting a children's yoga teacher certification. Having led guided imagery classes in Las Vegas and currently teaching three kids' yoga classes a week at my daughter's school, I have been a substitute teacher for the *very same healing yoga classes that brought me back to life, and I will soon be teaching children with cancer.*

The cancer survivors I have met are some of the happiest people I have ever known. They have formed a community of support and love and no one was scared of talking to me since they had all been down a similar path. They knew what it felt like to not be the person you were before and would never be again. We will always be cancer survivors and it has affected all of us.

Cancer decides when it comes back and what it feels like doing to us. It rules our lives and we need every tool we can find to fight it in ways that will support our mental happiness and our immune system. We need to be able to sleep and not be filled with anxiety, worry, and stress, or we will end up even sicker. I like to have a plan, but there is no plan. I will not know what cancer decides to do until it shows up on a CT scan or makes me sick enough to feel symptoms. It is the enemy and not even the doctors have a guarantee that they will be able to help me. I have a rare diagnosis, and there isn't even a proven medicine to help me if the cancer decided to grow. I have been given a five-year survival rate of 60 to 80 percent. So I might be at my daughter's tenth birthday or I might not. My breathing might deteriorate or it might not. I may need chemo or a lung transplant, or I might not.

Yoga has helped me to focus on what I know I can do. I can help other cancer survivors feel better through relaxing breathing exercises, guided visual-ization, yoga asanas, and the loving support of community. I was lucky to find the y4c training in New York City led by Tari Prinster. I was also pleasantly surprised when a young cancer survivor and fellow yoga teacher named Nancy, who I had previously met through a mutual friend, unrolled her yoga mat and sat down across from me in the very same teacher training. We had bonded through our cancer journey and now were on the same path to give back to this amazing community of survivors through yoga. When you have cancer you no longer feel part of normal society. It is like being exiled to Planet Cancer. It is extremely important to find other people like you who you can share your fears with as well as any advice on treatments or ways to cope with such strong feel-ings. That is why it is so crucial to have classes specifically for cancer survivors.

Yoga allows me to breathe. Yoga quiets my mind. Yoga allows me to move my body only as far as it should in that moment. Yoga has given me direction, a supportive community, and a way to share my joy of yoga with the world.

I am grateful for the gift of learning from Tari and the opportunity to share the teachings and joy of yoga with others. Namaste.

THE Y4C BUILDING BLOCKS

The y4c methodology has seven building blocks that are identifiable elements or phases of a recommended yoga practice. No matter how long you have been practicing or how strong your practice is, each element can be included and will ensure you are getting the most out of a yoga wellness plan. The building blocks are presented in a suggested sequence; however, the order is flexible—with an exception or two:

1. Dynamic Stillness: How to Sit
2. Pranayama: How to Breathe
3. Meditation: How to Quiet the Mind
4. Movement: How to Move with Ease
5. Balance: How to Build Focus, Bone, and Strength
6. Restorative Yoga: How to Actively Rest
7. Savasana: How to Seal It In

1. Dynamic Stillness: How to Sit

According to Swami Rama, "We are taught how to move and behave in the external world, but we are never taught how to be still and examine what is within ourselves. At the same time, learning to be still and calm should not be made a ceremony or part of any religion; it is a universal requirement of the human body."[2]

Your yoga practice starts with Dynamic Stillness. "Dynamic" means moving, while "stillness" means just the opposite. Even when we are sitting still with our bones comfortably settled, there is movement happening within the body. Our breath never stops expanding and contracting our lungs, our heart never stops pumping blood, our digestive system constantly absorbs and transports nutrients. All of the body's involuntary systems continue to function while we sit still. That is what is dynamic. The stillness is voluntary.

 Who you are is always changing, always opening, always breathing.

TARI PRINSTER

The act of sitting too is voluntary. When you think about it, the body is a container. The skin wraps around the architecture of the bones—the skeleton—which defines the size of the container. Inside are all the necessary parts, organs, and fluids to keep you alive. This is you. Where is that "container" right now? At this moment of beginning your yoga practice, your container is in that special space you have determined, or in a yoga class, sitting on a yoga mat or in a chair.

Becoming aware of where you are now may seem silly. But learning how to recognize this special feeling will bring you a profound understanding, serving as the start of your mind-body connection. You, in all your flesh and bones, are taking up space in the universe. Yes, the whole universe, in all its infiniteness.

When I think about this, it makes me feel both tiny and important. I feel tiny because of the vast reaches of space and time, but important too, because my finiteness is part of an infinite universe, if even for the tiny second of one small lifetime. To reflect, I need to sit and be still.

In yoga, we learn how to sit—how to place our bones within the framework of infinite space and time. Start by taking a seat on your yoga mat, as if you're at the center of the universe—which you are at this moment. You can also sit on a chair or stool, or on a bolster, cushion, or yoga block, cross-legged or with legs folded beneath you. It is important you find a position that is comfortable and stable enough that you can hold it for at least three minutes without fidgeting, shifting, or feeling any discomfort.

2. Pranayama: How to Breathe

Now that you have found your seat, you are ready to find and explore the first principle of y4c yoga, the breathing space, where you will quite literally learn how to breathe in a new way. In chapter 2, we learned why we need to focus on breathing, and how the breath nurtures and detoxifies our organs and cells, strengthening our immune system and keeping the body resistant to cancer. We also discussed the muscles used in creating the breath. The practice of doing yoga as a form of breathing is called *pranayama*, breath practice, or controlled breathing. With pranayama, you'll learn how to control, strengthen, and even enjoy the breath.

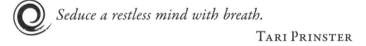 *Seduce a restless mind with breath.*

TARI PRINSTER

Breathing is simply the act of moving air. It creates a continuous supply of oxygen for cells to grow, heal, and stay alive. Muscles of the respiratory system move oxygen-rich air in and out of our lungs, so there is good reason to keep these muscles strong.

The breath movement has three parts: inhalation is the expansion that draws air into the lungs, exhalation is the contraction to push air out, and retention is the pause between inhaling and exhaling. It is here that we find stillness, using the respiratory muscles to hold air in or keep it out.

The exercises we will describe later in the book will strengthen the muscles that allow you to breathe and, in turn, increase your awareness and understanding of the breathing process. You will also enjoy the natural physical and mental relaxation that comes along with pranayama in a yoga practice.

3. Meditation: How to Quiet the Mind

Yoga teaches us to think differently and deeply about simple things in life like sitting and breathing. The same applies to how we use our minds. The word *meditation* has different meanings and misconceptions, the most common being that you just do it, and that directions are not necessary. Just like with breathing, most of us go through life thinking we do not need to learn anything about how to meditate, much less practice doing it. However, meditation involves much more than sitting still and blissing out.

Prior to my diagnosis, meditation did not come naturally to me. Perhaps I was too American in my thinking—always looking to my to-do list, distracted by the noisy world around.

Meditation is not another "something" to do. It requires learning to let go and it can't be forced. We have to learn how to be still. There is that word *still* again. It pops up almost as often as the word *practice*. Think about these words, use them, get comfortable with them.

 The Buddha does not close her eyes while meditating. She keeps them open to softly gaze at all life has to offer while staying focused on her spot.

TARI PRINSTER

Meditation is a gentle skill we want to learn, one that keeps the usual activities of the mind still, calm, and quiet. In other words, we are not thinking, not just doing "something," and that includes not sleeping.

Meditation is a practice in many religions and spiritual traditions. Here are a few interpretations of meditation:

- **Nothingness:** The practice of being in the moment, or as I like to call it, "brain laundry," the practice of keeping your mind clear of everything—thoughts, ideas, feelings. It is an active exercise that requires effort;

you're consciously using your mind to keep your thinking space clear of thoughts. This sounds easier than it is in practice, especially if you are new to meditation.

- **Watchfulness:** The practice of sitting and waiting to see what pops up, then observing that thought without reacting.
- **Exploration:** The practice of mentally traveling to a place with a specific thought, idea, or image in your mind, holding it and observing it.
- **Repetition:** The practice of whispering or mentally reciting a mantra or prayer is called *japa*.

Whether you are experienced or a beginner, each time you meditate stay with the intention, method, or tradition you chose that day. For new and experienced practitioners, it is expected that your mind will wander. That is what minds like to do. Thoughts come and thoughts go. Notice in that second and start over. It takes practice.

Meditation requires three things:

- A comfortable seated position
- A commitment to being curious about how it feels to not think. (I know this is hard, but it is where the healing happens.)
- The promise to yourself not to judge what comes up or happens. Observe and let go (catch and release).

Meditation is an essential survival tool for cancer survivors because we learn how to control, calm, and clear the mind of thoughts and ideas that are not useful. However, when practicing in a watchfulness tradition, for a cancer survivor, random thoughts can be frightening, not pleasant nor helpful to healing. Remember, you are in charge. If a scary thought presents itself, sweep it out with a breath, let it go. Watch your breath and let go of your thoughts. Cancer has already given us the "sit-down-let's-talk-about-the-here-and-now" lesson. Which means that *now* it is time to sit and meditate with the thought you choose or with your quiet and uncluttered mind.

Through meditation we gather strength to live well.
ANONYMOUS YOGA TEACHER

Finally, my students ask two questions about meditation.

• *How long should I meditate?*

Just like yoga, many different meditation techniques and styles exist. And just like yoga, meditation can be confusing. The types I recommend are simple, yet challenging. Even not thinking for just one minute requires effort and practice. It is a skill you can learn if you practice. For sure, the longer you practice, the more benefits you will experience. Length of time is not as important, though, as the quality of calmness you provide to the nervous system. Start with one minute, increasing that each time you practice. A daily five-minute meditation practice can have great benefits, like reduced anxiety and stress.

• *How often should I meditate?*

I think meditating twice a day is best. Let's add to the metaphor of meditation as brain laundry, meditation as mental hygiene. Do you not brush your teeth twice a day? Meditation is a great way to start the day. There is substantial research applying Mindfulness Based Stress Reduction (MBSR) to aid insomnia, which is a common side effect during many cancer treatments. The benefits of meditation before sleep is advised by sleep therapists for many chronic conditions.[3]

4. Movement: How to Move with Ease

A cancer survivor wants to keep the immune system healthy and alert. Many ways exist to maintain a strong system, but the most critical and natural way is through movement. By mobilizing muscles and bones, we massage the organs in our body that are otherwise inert. In fact, lack of movement can be as harmful as cancer. Movement improves circulation and mobilizes fluids like blood and lymph, which keep organ tissues nourished, and movement allows the body to detoxify. Movement keeps the body healthy. In his book *Light on Life,* renowned yoga teacher and author B. K. S. Iyengar says, "Movement is intelligent action."[4]

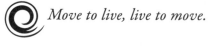 *Move to live, live to move.*

TARI PRINSTER

In the most basic sense, movement is created when muscles move bones. Taking this idea further, yoga uses muscles to place the bones into poses, or *asanas,* and then moves the body from pose to pose in sequences designed to bring all body systems into balance: muscles, bones, organs, and even the mind. Every cell in the body, the container that determines your real estate on Planet Earth, benefits from forming a yoga pose and moving in a sequence to other poses.

5. Balance: How to Build Focus, Bone, and Strength

Picture in your mind a Cirque du Soleil performer: Her perfect sculptured body is tiny and flexible, a model of a healthy young athlete. One at a time, she places a foot on the shoulders of her partner. Then, in what seems like a seamless movement, she lifts her left foot to that perfect spot on her partner's head. Like a bird taking flight, she rises onto the tippy-toe of her ballet slipper. All of her weight is balanced six feet above the ground atop a moving, breathing person!

Finding balance is a life's work.

TARI PRINSTER

Yes, this is a circus act, but we all do this every day when we place one foot in front of the next, walking down the street. We're moving, breathing objects balancing ourselves on another moving object, Earth. Like the circus performer, our body systems need to be working together to carry us through life. This is part of the balance we find in our yoga practice. Like the circus performer, we need to practice balance, and yoga poses help us do just that.

Of course, it's hard enough to stay balanced on two feet sometimes, so why would you need or want to try balancing on one foot? There are many answers—and they're all simple:

- Challenging your balance tests your connection to the Earth. This can only be done when there is harmony between your thoughts and body.
- Practicing balance poses increases your ability to focus. When this happens, it is easier to do the same when it comes to the other things in life that are important.
- Weight-bearing exercise strengthens bones.
- Good balance helps protect you from falling and breaking bones.
- Good balance improves your posture, which helps you breathe.
- Overall, practicing balancing keeps the immune system well.

You may wonder why so many yoga poses are performed on one foot, like the feats of a circus performer. One-foot poses teach us proper alignment of the spine and how to use the act of weight bearing to build bone. Correct alignment comes from knowledge and practice. When we are aligned, we use the strong bones of our body's frame to hold our weight. We learn that standing on one foot on our moving planet becomes easier.

Alignment makes balancing easier but so does breathing. This is the second way yoga teaches us balance. In doing balance poses, no matter how easy, let your effort be supported by your breath. I am sure you have noticed how a relaxed person enjoying a quiet moment does not breathe like a runner finishing a 100-meter race. You've also never seen an anxious person breathe deeply, slowly, and with ease. So, breath quality—whether hard, calm, fast, slow, shallow, or deep—is the first and obvious indication of our state of mind and well-being.

 Life is all about balance. Since I have only one leg, I understand that well.

SANDY FUSSELL

The mind follows the breath. A calm breath will support your balance poses in a physical way, while practicing simple balancing yoga poses will train your body and mind to work together to stay balanced. Staying upright on one foot in Tree pose for thirty seconds may not be easy, for example, but a lesson is found in this state of mental and physical harmony. When the mind and body work together, we are calm and balanced.

This is why balancing is good for cancer patients. Call this mental focus or strength: it is healing to know how to clear your body and mind of anxious moments by standing on one foot! With the exception of lying on our backs, just about every yoga pose requires keeping bones properly placed through the use of our muscles, and supporting that with an easy breath. Balance is required even when standing on two feet or on all fours. Right here, right now.

6. Restorative Yoga: How to Actively Rest

Restorative poses have great benefits when used at the end of your practice to close and seal in the hard work you have completed. As you follow the restorative poses in my book, you'll notice they feel magical because we are surprised by the changes we experience. That magic, though, is based on scientific research that led to the development of restorative yoga, which means "resting with purpose." When practicing restorative poses you're literally restoring balance in your body's architecture, organ functions, and mind.

Restorative yoga uses props like blocks, blankets, and bolsters to completely support your body—so you can literally "take a load off" and reduce stress. (Your only movement will be when you arrange the props and get into the pose.) The props not only release you of effort, but also position your body in such a way so as to reduce strain on joints. Your body can completely relax into stillness. As it does, the mind relaxes into stillness too and grows calm and quiet.

Most restorative poses are done lying down, and the body is placed in one of the five spinal positions that are the foundation of every yoga style: elongation, forward (flexion), back (extension), side bends, and twists. Here is where the magic begins: when the body's architecture (skeleton) is properly aligned (especially the spine), effort evaporates and deep rest begins.

Earlier, we observed this process in the "Dynamic Stillness" (pages 92–93) and "Meditation" (pages 94–96) sections. Here though, the goal is total relaxation: the state in which there is no movement, no effort, no muscles holding bones. (This is different than a sitting pose, for example, in which the spine needs to be upright, with ribs stacked on hips, shoulders broad, neck lifted, and head balanced atop the spine.)

The poses can be sustained for ten minutes or more as long as you remain comfortable and are still experiencing the magic. Deep, delicious rest is just one reason why restorative yoga poses are so popular. What's more, all the benefits of regular yoga are achieved without effort.

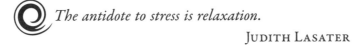

The antidote to stress is relaxation.

JUDITH LASATER

Finally, I want to say more about cancer and restorative yoga. We know cancer increases stress. But what exactly is stress? It is a term borrowed from physics and engineering that, when applied to humans, describes a psychological state. When a building's structure or foundation is under stress, there is danger of collapse. Likewise, when the human body is weakened by lack of proper care, nurture, and nutrients; injury; disease; or immune system failure, stress is created.

When it comes to yoga, stress is a very good reason for survivors to include restorative poses in every yoga practice. Restorative yoga nourishes the entire body and its systems. Most importantly, a strong immune system is achieved when all the body's systems find balance and work in harmony.

Relaxing is a nervous system response to the special placement of the spine in different positions, and it rejuvenates the musculoskeletal system. When combined with breathing exercises, the respiratory system gets stimulated. Even gentle movement of the breath revitalizes the digestive organs and stimulates the endocrine system. So, all aspects of the immune system are involved in every restorative pose.

Cultivating attention and focusing on the breath are two other goals of restorative yoga. When the mind wanders during these poses, you are encouraged to think about how your breath is moving in and out. This is the only movement allowed! Each exhale is an opportunity to release distracting thoughts as well as muscle tension.

The body's capacity to heal itself is infinite, and for most of one's life it does this well. Deep relaxation starts inside, just like healing, and it comes from within. The more you relax, the more peaceful you become, and the more healing you give yourself.

We have another magical benefit from restorative yoga. Our bodies and moods change every day. Restorative yoga is wonderful if included after more vigorous, energizing movement and balance sequences, but it could also be done on its own, depending on your mood or feeling that day. This may be appropriate at some stages of cancer recovery. Having a balance of both movement and rest in our daily lives is what keeps us strong and healthy.

7. Savasana: How to Seal It In

Savasana is the bliss spot in a yoga practice and its most important ingredient. For this pose you simply rest comfortably with your back flat on your mat, arms slightly away from the body with hands open to the sky. The ultimate goal of Savasana is sealing in all your work on the mat from the other poses. Your restorative poses paved the way, and this last pose completes your practice.

Don't be alarmed: the word *Savasana* is Sanskrit for Corpse pose. It has alternate names, all of which describe its corpse-like posture: deep relaxation pose, final resting pose, and in the y4c method, Sunset pose.

Sunset pose, as I refer to it, may not seem like much, but it's the most essential pose of a yoga practice, especially for cancer patients and survivors. In fact, this pose is the ultimate restorative pose that is always at the end of your session and should never be skipped. Like all restorative poses, Sunset pose uses no muscular effort, no thinking, and no moving.

Few if any props are used. If you are cold, you can cover yourself with a blanket to keep warm. If you experience discomfort in your back, you can place a rolled blanket or bolster under your knees.

Sunset pose incorporates a natural breath. It is complete and utter relaxation. Even so, it might just be the hardest pose to perform in your practice. At least it was for me.

When I restarted my yoga practice during and after cancer treatments, I found Sunset pose difficult and scary. Difficult, not because I could not do it, but because I could not get physically comfortable. Something was always in pain: my back, my hips, my joints. Once I realized where and how to place folded blankets beneath my legs and back, and stopped judging myself for not being able to relax, the lingering muscle tension eased.

Several months of shifting and experimenting were necessary. Teaching the body to relax is not easy, nor is it fast. In my case, my mind was the problem! My brain kept sending signals based on muscle memory to hold myself tightly and not release, sending the message, "Things are not quite right. I am still working." Once my bones were supported by soft blankets, muscles released and sent signals to my mind with the message, "I don't need to keep working. I'm okay. Let's both relax."

Now, with many years of yoga experience, I quickly find that bliss spot. This is the "letting go" that yoga teachers talk about. My muscle memory is programmed through practice to alert my brain to the good things to come. Ah, ten minutes of relaxation! In short, like any other yoga pose, Sunset pose takes practice. We have to learn how to do it.

 Sometimes it's those things we least understand that deserve our deepest trust.

PICO IYER

If the monkeys in your mind start swinging in the trees, hang in there. For cancer patients and survivors, there are many things we do not like to see, inside and out, and worries could pop up during Sunset pose, bringing unwanted stress and making it harder to achieve conscious rest. Tense muscles and joint pain could accompany these thoughts, making the resting pose more anxiety-inducing than healing. Meditation can help calm your mind so your body can heal. Here are other ways to tame the monkeys that distract us:

- Learn how to make yourself comfortable using blankets to support your body.
- Accept the precious gift of time to heal. It's not expensive to be still in the mind and body.
- Imagine the sunset as you perform the sunset of the day's yoga practice. It's okay if you bliss out, or even fall asleep. Try not to sleep, but if you do, accept the rest as a gift to yourself.

Remember: Everything has a cycle, be it a single breath, a life, a human cell, or a yoga practice. Everything has a beginning, middle, and end point. As things begin to end, the anticipation of the new beginning arises. The natural closing of each day with a sunset is necessary to make way for the next sunrise. There's no need to rush. Use this time—your time—to heal and restore.

*Start with doing
what is necessary,
consider trying what is
possible, and suddenly
you find yourself doing
the impossible.*

SAINT FRANCIS OF ASSISI

Veronica, cancer survivor

5

Preparing for Your Practice

I gave the room a once over, which was all it deserved. Fluorescent lights flickered above desk chairs lined up on a dirty linoleum floor. The hospital must have used this room for workshops and seminars. But for my purposes it wouldn't do. How on earth, I thought, could a cancer survivor take a yoga class on a dirty linoleum floor in the foot-and-a-half of space between two rows of desk chairs? How could anyone, for that matter, feel comfortable taking a yoga class here?

Sure, this clinic was willing to offer yoga classes, but it lacked the tools and resources to create an appropriate, safe, and comfortable environment. Everything—from the desk chairs to the dirty floor—suggested that the class came about because someone simply said, "We've heard this yoga stuff is good. We'll provide a space and a time, but that's it. . . ."

Today was my first day teaching at the clinic, and the janitor had set up folding chairs on which many of the women had already taken a seat. Apparently, the yoga that had been taught here before had been done entirely while seated in chairs.

"These won't be necessary," I said to the janitor, eyeing the chairs. "Would you mind putting them back?"

Instantly, the palpable resistance in the room melted away. When these women realized they were not going to be sitting in chairs and treated like sick people, and that they were actually going to sit on the floor and do yoga, the entire room breathed a sigh of relief and tittered with excitement.

Fortunately, the clinic did have yoga mats and blankets handy. After showing my new students how to spread their mats on the floor and fold their blankets, we were ready to begin.

CREATING THE RIGHT SPACE AND TIME FOR YOGA

When beginning a yoga practice or getting back into it after a cancer diagnosis, a few basic steps will get you going. Constructing a yoga practice is like building a house: you start with a location, building materials, tools, and a set of plans to create and maintain it. Of course, a good carpenter is helpful too. In crafting a yoga practice, that builder is you. Let's get started.

Step 1. Choose Your Yoga Space

As evident in the clinic story, space is an important concept when it comes to yoga: Where you choose to practice is so important. You may practice at a clinic, health club, yoga studio, or at home.

If you are going to do yoga at home, find a spot that is unencumbered. You should be able to move freely, without touching objects around you, like the coffee table or couch. Imagine a 5 x 7-foot area as your minimum. Your yoga space should also be quiet, private, and comfortable. Much like the location you'd choose for building a new home, your yoga space is literally the real estate for a very important project: you.

Step 2. Find Your Yoga Time

There's another type of space you'll need to get started: time in your calendar to spend just on yourself! This "time space" is not easy to carve out in a busy life. Creating the time for yoga is just as important as finding the physical space or venue. Here are five ways to squeeze precious, private minutes into your day.

- Manage interruptions by scheduling yoga much like you would a lunch date, doctor's appointment, or business meeting. That way you can tell family and friends you have a meeting planned and can't be disturbed, even if your meeting is with yourself!

- Mark your yoga class on all your calendars, including the one on your mobile device.
- Turn off the TV and the ringer on your cell phone so that you're free of distractions. Clean out the noise clutter, fill the room with quiet.
- Close the door to your space, if that's possible. It's important to have your own private space.
- Soft music is fine. This also signals to others that you are taking time for your yoga practice.

Creating this time for yourself is a life skill, one that extends beyond cancer recovery. In this way, yoga can aid your time management practice, along with all aspects of life. Time management is essential during cancer treatment, healing, and your continued recovery. Cultivating support within your environment—from your family and friends—is key and is part of your job as a survivor. Let the people in your life know you need to have this space and time, and give it to yourself. It is *your* time and you need to claim it.

Step 3. Prepare Your Tool Kit

If you want to cook a fabulous meal you need the proper materials, like sturdy pots, utensils, and even tasty spices. In yoga, the materials you need are called *props*. At minimum, you should have a yoga sticky mat. Proper yoga mats are no more than a half-inch thick and feature a slip-resistant surface. (See pages 111–14 for more on yoga props.)

Often, gyms have extra-thick mats because it is thought that more cushioning is better, especially if you are experiencing discomfort—whether cancer-related or not. Actually, less cushioning is better, and gives you more control over your poses. Too much cushioning can make it harder to balance and even cause injury.

You will need at least two yoga blocks, which can be purchased at any sporting goods store, and two to four soft blankets. A specially made yoga bolster and a yoga strap are helpful, but not essential. You can also roll a blanket to double as a bolster. All these props will help tailor your practice according to your specific physical needs.

Almost all yoga poses in this book can be done from a chair, so if you feel you could use extra support, then a chair is great. (Examples of how to use the chair in different poses will be provided in chapter 6.) The chair should be placed on a yoga mat to prevent it from slipping on the floor.

Many poses can also be done from a bed or couch. These modifications are noted in chapter 6 and can be applied to the gentle sample practices in chapter 7.

Step 4. Create Your Yoga Practice

In constructing my personal yoga practice, I use the building blocks discussed in chapter 4 (pages 92–101) that are essential for healing. They provide the formula for constructing your practice each time you visit your mat.

Each section of this book was written with the overall goal of balancing all the body's systems. Although presented in order, the poses and sequences in chapters 6 and 7 are flexible and customizable, taking into account what you may be dealing with in terms of cancer and other special conditions. Together they create a complete practice that matches your needs.

Unlike a doctor who practices medicine, or a baseball player who practices with her team, a yoga practice is more like personal hygiene for the body and the mind. Please be kind to yourself; you may not feel the same way every day. Every day is different. One day you'll wake up cranky. Another day, you feel like Wonder Woman. Because of this, your yoga practice should not be the same. That would get terribly boring, and it's healthier to add variety—just like it is good to change up your salads so you can benefit from different vitamins found within varied ingredients. Yoga is a perfect match for the challenges of treating and surviving cancer because the poses are so adaptable.

The fifty-three yoga poses in this book will be your ingredients for creating a personalized yoga practice in which you can select the poses that create a practice to meet your daily needs. Like a good meal, your practice should nurture all the body's systems.

We've already discussed practicing yoga on a daily basis. But what about the actual amount of time you should dedicate to your practice? As with all prescriptions, dosage depends on the individual—except in this case, it's one step better: you can formulate your yoga practice based on how you feel.

Here are guidelines to follow.

- Ask your doctor if it is safe for you to do gentle exercise. The answer may not be related to your cancer, but perhaps even to other medical conditions. Follow what's best and safest for you.
- If you've had surgery, drains must be removed before practicing yoga. Chemotherapy ports, however, if properly healed, are safe.
- You are the carpenter of your yoga experience. Listen to your body and adapt your practice to its changes. Are you tired? sore? energized? Let your body speak!

Remember: yoga has the flexibility to adapt to you, and not the other way around.

Chapter 7 features several sample practices from which you can pick and choose, or even combine to create your own. Your goal is to build a yoga practice that you want to do every day—because your body would miss it otherwise! And when doing yoga becomes like physical and mental hygiene, then it becomes a practice—just like brushing your teeth. Of course, how often you do yoga is only a matter of how often you can. If it makes you feel good and look good, why would you not do it every day?

*I don't like to gamble,
but if there's one thing
I'm willing to bet on,
it's myself.*

BEYONCÉ

Michelle, cancer survivor

6

Creating Your Yoga Practice and Learning the Poses

Yoga poses for cancer patients and survivors are not much different than those for everyone else: we all need strong immune systems, muscles moving, fluids flowing! The poses in this book, however, have been selected for their specific benefits to target what the survivor most needs.

Not all yoga poses may be beneficial for cancer survivors. Some popular poses should be avoided or used only with great caution. All poses have benefits and potential risks, especially if used in the wrong way. Here are the "ABCs" for choosing the right pose: *awareness*, *benefits*, and *common sense*.

AWARENESS

Be aware of your physical health, restrictions, and limitations, whether related to cancer or not. If you had physical problems like arthritis or high blood pressure before being diagnosed with cancer, it's likely you still have them. Our other problems do not go away; cancer does not eliminate other health problems. Whether temporary or chronic, they should not be ignored. If viewed in a holistic way, one condition affects all conditions. The body awareness we develop in yoga can be a tool to identify what the body is feeling. You can learn to identify whether an uncomfortable feeling or sensation you have is caused by arthritis, or by stiffness from sleeping in a new bed; this is a part of putting together your personal yoga plan.

When it comes to cancer, awareness and attention to health conditions and treatment side effects will affect how you choose your poses and level of activity. And you should be mindful of any benefits and risks. For example, care should be taken with surgical drains, as these are open wounds and could be a source of infection. I would recommend that you wait until they are removed before starting a yoga program. However, a chemo port (a catheter or port-a-cath placed beneath the skin and used for chemotherapy infusions) is usually not a problem if properly healed. But it's helpful for your teacher to know if you have one and where it is. Do not hesitate or be embarrassed to communicate this information. Your teacher will be grateful and careful. Also, after a chemo port is removed—reason to celebrate—there may be residual scar tissue as well as a tightness that limits movement. Restricted movement can cause, over time, imbalances unrelated to cancer or a preexisting condition. Again, be aware, not alarmed.

Awareness also is required by your teacher. If you are attending yoga classes, be sure to inform your teacher of your body conditions and any sensitive parts of your body. This will ensure the safest and most effective practice.

BENEFITS

Yoga is a tool of empowerment—an ability to control your own recovery plan. For you to best "prescribe" what you need means that you have to know the benefits of the poses, sequences, and practices. On one day you might feel strong and want to build strength, burn calories, and improve your flexibility. On another day, perhaps after a chemotherapy appointment, you might want to do some detoxifying twists with some relaxing restorative poses. To make this easier, I have included the specific benefits and modifications of each pose so you can tailor them to your particular needs. This will help guide your choices depending on your goals, such as cardiovascular fitness, building bone density, or weight management.

COMMON SENSE

Without discounting the knowledge of your doctors, you know your body and mind best. As a yoga teacher, I can guide you into the pose with my words and hands, but I cannot know exactly what you feel. In fact, no teacher can tell you if a yoga pose feels bad unless they know what you bring to the yoga mat. So, it's important to use common sense when performing yoga; know your physical limits and what feels right for you. If you are in class, you should communicate your concerns to your teacher.

Now here's the most important part: enjoy! Enjoy your yoga. Let it help you feel good about your body. Let's get started.

In the section below, fifty-three unique poses are provided that are tailored to the specific needs of a cancer patient and survivor. Each pose is accompanied by an instructive illustration and description along with any benefits and modifications. Some of them have been grouped by *vinyasa*—a Sanskrit term that simply refers to a sequence of poses that link movement with breath. My recommendation is that you fully review all these poses to better understand what options you have. Chapter 7 includes sequences of poses based on exertion level and time length (thirty, sixty, or ninety minutes). Chapter 8 includes poses designed to address particular side effects (such as lymphedema, bone loss, weight gain, anxiety, etc.).

When it comes to cancer, lingering effects are often not mentioned. When it comes to yoga, lingering effects are the reason to do it.

TARI PRINSTER

GETTING READY—PROPS

Yoga props were originally introduced in the twentieth century by B. K. S. Iyengar in order to support proper physical alignment and prevent injury. Props can be useful to practitioners of all levels, from beginner to advanced students, as tools to assist in developing stability, flexibility, ease, and relaxation. Common props include yoga mats, blankets, blocks, bolsters, and straps.

Yoga Mat

Yoga mats, usually made of textured rubber or PVC, provide comfort, stability, safety, and steadiness by ensuring your feet and hands won't slip during practice, and the mat won't slide on the floor. Mats come in varying degrees of thickness, which provides a cushion between your body and the ground. However, there is a trade-off between comfort and stability when choosing the thickness of your mat. A thinner mat means a firmer connection to the ground. Too much cushioning will make balancing difficult.

Don't have a yoga mat? A yoga mat is highly recommended, particularly if you plan to practice standing and balancing poses. However if you don't have a yoga mat, you can also use a nonslip yoga towel on top of a rug. An exercise mat is not a good alternative, as they are generally much thicker than yoga mats, and tend to be slippery.

Yoga Blanket

A yoga blanket can be folded into various sizes and shapes for specialized support, or used for warmth. The yoga blanket is a multifaceted tool for supporting the alignment of the body and providing extra cushioning, particularly for the knees, hips, neck, and shoulders. A blanket may help you perform poses that might otherwise be overly challenging or uncomfortable due to lack of range of motion or flexibility. It can help keep your body in balance if one side is less mobile than the other, and encourages relaxation.

Don't have a yoga blanket? You can use any blanket of substantial thickness and size. Towels are generally too thin to be a good substitute.

Yoga Block

The yoga block, usually made of foam, wood, or cork, is a solid, rectangular object designed to support the weight of your body for improved stability, alignment, and ease.

It serves as an extension of your body to the floor. For instance, blocks are often used under the hands in standing poses so the hands can be supported on a stable, flat surface if they can't reach the ground. Blocks can improve body alignment and create extension in the spine, provide support during balancing poses, and help you move safely in and out of a posture.

Don't have a yoga block? You can also use a stack of books, a chair, or the hands of a helping friend. Ensure your support structure is stable enough to take your weight, and the correct height that you need.

Yoga mat

Yoga blankets

Yoga blankets

Bolster

Strap

Eye pillow

Yoga blocks

Yoga Bolster

The yoga bolster is a large, firm pillow, usually cylindrical or rectangular in shape, used to support your body weight so you can experience the benefits of a yoga pose without exerting effort. Most often used in restorative poses, the bolster promotes complete relaxation. It is firm enough to hold your body in a posture while encouraging deep muscular release.

Don't have a yoga bolster? You can use a narrow couch cushion, a stack of firm pillows, or several folded blankets.

Yoga Strap

The yoga strap, usually six to eight feet long, with a buckle on one end, connects one part of the body to another for an intensified stretch, improved alignment, or deeper relaxation. It can help the body move into a pose more effectively, while achieving correct posture with less effort. It can help you learn challenging poses by moving into them incrementally, for instance, by artificially adding length to your arms and allowing you to stretch to your own range of motion and not strain beyond. The strap can also bind together parts of the body, stabilizing one area in order to mobilize or relax another.

Don't have a yoga strap? You can use the belt of a bathrobe, a necktie, or any strap made of material that is smooth and durable so as not to be abrasive.

STARTING YOUR PRACTICE

Taking Your Seat

Begin your yoga practice by taking your seat and finding stillness. You can sit in a chair or on the floor in a position that is comfortable and supports your spine to be fully upright. This will allow you to effectively practice meditation, breathing (pranayama), and many warm-up sequences. You can switch your seated posture at any time, and start each practice differently. The more you develop stability in your seated position, the easier it becomes to cultivate centered stillness of the body and mind.

In order to cultivate your physical stability, visualize your body in the shape of a pyramid—wide and grounded at the base and well-supported as it rises to the topmost point, the crown of your head. Part of the reason ancient pyramids were designed in this way was to symbolize the royal footprint left on the earth by a king or queen. So sit regally, your seat a throne and your body a pyramid.

TAKING YOUR SEAT IN A CHAIR

Props needed: Chair

Sit upright in a sturdy chair, placing your feet flat on the floor beneath your knees, hip distance apart.

Modifications: Place blocks or cushions under your feet if they do not reach the floor.

Benefits: Body awareness, breath awareness, spinal alignment, focusing the mind, relaxation

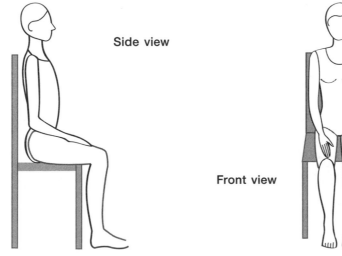

Side view

Front view

TAKING YOUR SEAT IN A CROSS-LEGGED POSITION

Props needed: Blankets or cushion

Sit on blankets or a cushion, crossing your shins. Make these supports high enough that your knees are level with, or below, your hips. This makes it easier to sit fully upright and to breathe more freely. If your hips or inner thighs feel strained, place yoga blocks or blankets under your knees for extra support.

Modifications: If one knee is higher than the other, support both knees with props at the height required so that both knees are level and your body remains symmetrical. If you have hip or knee pain, try extending one or both legs out in front of you.

Benefits: Body awareness, breath awareness, spinal alignment, focusing the mind, relaxation

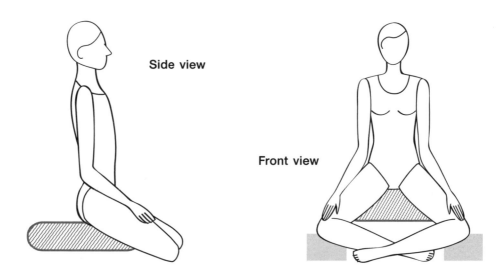

Side view

Front view

TAKING YOUR SEAT IN VIRASANA—HERO POSE

Props needed: Blankets, blocks, or cushions

Spread a blanket on your mat or the floor. Kneel on the blanket with the tops of your feet resting on the floor and place a block, cushion, or folded blanket between your feet. Settle your hips on this support, bringing your knees close together.

Modifications: If this pose is uncomfortable for your knees, ankles, or feet, try elevating your hips higher with an additional yoga block, blanket, or cushion. To relieve pressure in the ankles and tops of the feet, place a small rolled-up blanket under each ankle.

Benefits: Body awareness, breath awareness, spinal alignment, focusing the mind, relaxation

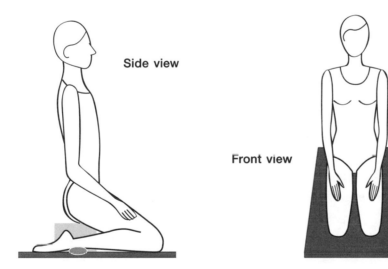

Side view

Front view

118

How to Build
Your Own
Yoga Practice

•

Finding
Dynamic Stillness

Finding Dynamic Stillness

Whether you are sitting in a chair or on the floor cross-legged or in Hero pose, find the proper, neutral alignment for your spine and begin to find stillness.

Your pelvis is shaped like a bowl. At the bottom of the bowl are your two sitting bones. Rock your hips from side to side in your seat until you feel your weight evenly balanced between your right and left sitting bone. Then tilt the bowl of your pelvis forward and back. Notice that when you are slightly forward on your sitting bones your spine is at its full height. Maintain this position as the stable base of your neutral spine. Feel the bones of your spine stacking from this base of support to hold you effortlessly upright.

. . . .

DYNAMIC STILLNESS

Center the crown of your head over your hips, chin parallel to the floor.

Place your hands on your thighs in a position in which your elbows rest directly below your shoulders.

With a soft gaze, let your eyes rest on the floor about six feet in front of you.

INHALE: Lengthen your spine, broadening your shoulders.

EXHALE: Distribute weight evenly into your seat, maintaining an upright spine.

Benefits: Body awareness, breath awareness, spinal alignment, focusing the mind, relaxation

 If you are able to quiet your mind to hear your breath and heartbeat, a healing process unfolds that is life preserving.

Tari Prinster

Taking Time to Breathe

Developing breath awareness will focus your mind and support your body as you cultivate your yoga practice. Begin each practice with a few minutes of simple breathing. I have included several exercises to choose from.

At the start of any of these breathing exercises, take a few moments to notice your natural, unaltered breath. Observe your habitual breathing patterns. What parts of your body expand and contract as you breathe? Does your breath feel shallow or deep, rough or smooth? Do you usually breathe through your nose or your mouth?

During the breathing practices and yoga sequences that follow, it is preferable to breathe in and out through your nose, if possible. As you start to control your breathing and use specific techniques, do so with a light touch, so your breath can remain calm and without strain. At first it may feel uncomfortable to control or even simply observe your breathing. Stay with a breathing exercise for a few breaths, then rest and breathe normally, noticing if the exercise has affected your normal breathing patterns. You may repeat the exercise two or three times, with short breaks in between for observation.

EQUAL BREATH

Sit in the dynamic stillness posture of your choice. As you observe your breath, notice if your inhales are shorter or longer than your exhales. Begin to assign a length to your breath by silently counting as you breathe—Inhale one, two, three . . . exhale one, two, three. Use your counting to make your inhales and exhales an equal length. Adjust the speed of your counting to match the natural length of your breath, so you can breathe with the least possible effort. As you practice, you may be able to increase the count to four counts for the inhale and four counts for the exhale. Continue to lengthen your breath by adding to the count if you can do so without strain.

120

How to Build
Your Own
Yoga Practice

Taking Time
to Breathe

SMILING BUDDHA EYES

Sit in dynamic stillness. Focus your eyes on a single point in front of you. Relax your facial muscles. As you inhale, without moving your head or your eyes, expand your gaze so you take in the entire space in front of you and in your peripheral vision. As you exhale narrow your focus back to the singular point you have chosen. With each inhale expand your gaze as wide as you can with soft eyes. With each exhale make your focus singular and directed. Keep your breathing easy and natural.

BELLY BUTTON BREATH

Lie on your back in a restful position. You can bend your knees and place your feet on the floor, or rest your knees over a bolster or rolled blanket, adding a small pillow under your head for optimal comfort. Place a lightweight yoga block (not a heavy wooden one) on your belly, right on top of your belly button (you can also use a small cushion or book). Rest your arms by your sides. As you inhale notice how your belly rises, lifting the block. As you exhale your belly falls with the weight of the block. Keeping your belly relaxed, see if with each inhale you can lift the block slightly higher, and by exhaling more completely you can sink the block more deeply. Move the block with your breath, not your abdominal muscles.

THREE-PART BREATH: BEGINNING, MIDDLE, END

Lie on your back in a restful position with supportive props, as you did for Belly Button Breath. Place your hands on your belly, palms down. Feel your breath under your hands. In this exercise, your inhales will remain natural. Your exhales will be broken into three parts. Begin by taking a full inhale. Exhale one-third of your breath out and pause, holding your breath. Continue exhaling another third of your breath out and pause. Complete your exhale, emptying out your breath and pause. Allow your inhale to pour into your body without effort. Rest for three natural breaths, then repeat the exercise.

A Moment of Meditation

Taking time to breathe can lead quite naturally into a moment of meditation. To begin, sit in dynamic stillness. You can also meditate lying down, standing, or walking, but a comfortable, upright seat is an ideal physical container to develop a wakeful, relaxed mental state. Lying down often makes the mind sleepy, therefore making meditation more challenging.

While taking time to breathe you may have already noticed how easily distracted the mind is, jumping from one thought to the next like a monkey jumping from branch to branch. The Buddha called this "monkey mind." In meditation we begin to tame our monkey mind, first by choosing a point of focus. Your focal point can be your breathing, a visualization, a mantra (a meaningful word or phrase you repeat silently to yourself), or a guided journey. I offer here a few different approaches to creating your own personal moment of meditation, which might be just a minute or two, or longer as your concentration and time allows.

Bringing your awareness to your natural, unaltered breath is always a good place to start. You may choose to close your eyes or with a soft, steady gaze keep them focused on a point on the floor about three feet in front of you. As you observe your breath, you will notice your thoughts begin to wander. Each time your mind wanders away, gently and without judgment bring your focus back to your breath. Or, if it is helpful, bring your focus back to the mantra words or your chosen visual image. Let this be your guide. No matter the state in which you find your mind, be kind to yourself. This is a practice of self-acceptance.

When we feel troubled by a difficult emotional state, we can become useful and activate our healing process by tapping in to our capacity to create positive emotions guided by positive thoughts. Here are some suggestions of simple healing mantras and visual guides.

. . . .

PEACE PLEASE

Repeat silently to yourself—

As you inhale: *I fill with peace and ease.*
As you exhale: *I let go of what I do not need.*

122

How to Build
Your Own
Yoga Practice
•
A Moment
of Meditation

CLOUDLESS SKY

Imagine your mind is a clear sky, wide and blue. Your thoughts are clouds in the sky. Notice as the clouds arise and let them drift away, returning to the empty blue sky, returning your attention to your breath.

SURFING THE WAVES

Visualize your inhale as a wave rising to its white crest. Imagine your exhale as the foaming, frothing water tumbling down onto the sandy beach. This may be the best surfing day all year. Ride the waves.

JOURNEY OF THE SENSES

Begin this self-guided journey by visualizing yourself in your ideal place: a lush forest, a mountaintop, a tropical beach, an open field. . . . Wake up all your senses. Smell the air. Feel the rock, the sand, the grass, or the touch of your clothing. Taste the breeze, salty or sweet. Hear the birds, the waves, the music. Let the world around you unfold. Be fully present.

MOVING MEDITATION

This meditation is distinct from the others as it is practiced while walking. Usually when we walk, our focus is on where we are going. In walking meditation, the focus is on the act of walking itself. You can practice this while walking down the street, or in a circle around your living room. Focus your attention on the physical sensation of your feet meeting the ground. Optionally, you can also add a breath focus or a mantra. Lift your foot slowly as you inhale—heel, ball, toe. Place the foot down as you exhale—heel, ball, toe. Or repeat silently as you inhale: Walking this way, and as you exhale: I am grateful for today. Walk into the present moment.

 From your seat of choice, take the first step into your practice. Then take a moment of meditation.

TARI PRINSTER

GETTING WARMED UP

Starting to Move with Your Breath

PELVIC TILT

Sit upright with hands on your hips. Use your hands to bring awareness to the movement of the hips in this sequence.

INHALE: Rock to the front of your sitting bones, moving the front of your hips toward your thighs to arch your spine. Lift your chest and draw your elbows behind you.

EXHALE: Rock to the back of your sitting bones, rounding your spine. Let your head fall forward as you pull your belly back. Elbows move out to the sides.

Repeat sequence five times.

Benefits: Breath awareness, coordinates movement with breath, spine mobility, hip flexibility, chest opening, releases neck tension, releases tension in upper and lower back

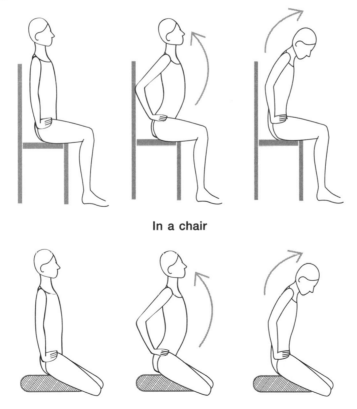

In a chair

In a cross-legged position

124

How to Build
Your Own
Yoga Practice

•

Starting to Move
with Your Breath

NECK STRETCH

Begin in your upright seat with your head balanced on top of your spine, chin parallel with the floor.

INHALE: Lengthen your spine, sitting tall.

EXHALE: Slowly lean your right ear toward your right shoulder. Relax the muscles on the left side of your neck.

INHALE: Reach your left hand actively toward the floor beside your left hip, turning your left hand so the palm faces forward and then away from you.

EXHALE: Gently lean your head a little bit further to the right to increase the stretch.

INHALE: Bring your head back upright

EXHALE: Lean your head to the right, into the stretch.

Repeat the last two steps for five breaths. Then switch to the second side, leaning left ear toward left shoulder while reaching the right hand toward the floor.

Modifications: This sequence can also be done standing.

Benefits: Breath awareness; coordinates movement with breath; releases neck, shoulder, and upper back tension

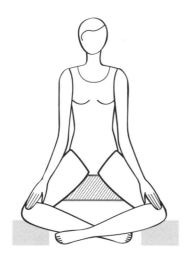 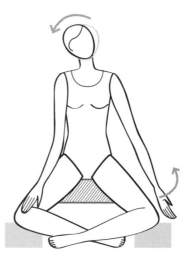

GATHER AND HOLD

In a seated position, rest the backs of your hands on your thighs or any appropriate surface with your fingers curled in toward your palms.

INHALE for a count of three, opening your fingers wide as if to receive a gift. EXHALE for a count of three while curling your fingers back in to your palms.

Repeat for five to ten breaths.

Modifications: If you can, lengthen your inhales and exhales by adding more counts to the breath. If your breath feels strained, shorten the count.

Benefits: Breath awareness, coordinates movement with breath, focuses the mind, relaxation

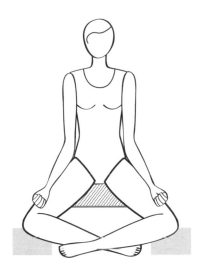
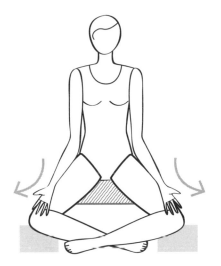

Arm Vinyasas

THUMBS-UP

Sit upright, reaching your arms toward the floor on either side of you without touching the floor, thumbs pointing down.

INHALE: Turn your thumbs to point away from you by rotating your upper arms, not just your wrists. Feel your shoulders and shoulder blades as part of this movement. As your shoulder blades move toward each other your chest opens.

EXHALE: Turn your thumbs to point down again, using the rotation of your whole arm and movement of the shoulders.

Repeat sequence five times.

Benefits: Range of motion in shoulders and arms, chest and upper back stretch, lymphatic drainage in arms

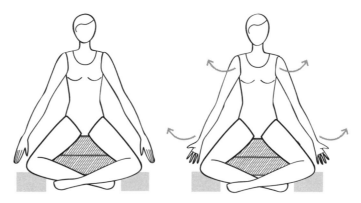

Front view

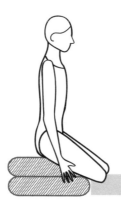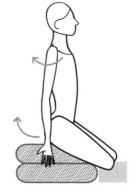

Side view

CACTUS CLAP

Sit upright with palms on your thighs.

INHALE: Lift your arms to shoulder height, bending your elbows to make a cactus shape, with palms facing forward.

EXHALE: Bring your palms and forearms together in front of your face.

INHALE: Reopen your arms to Cactus. Move slowly, following your breath.

Repeat the last two steps three times. Then lower your arms and rest your palms on your thighs.

Modifications: Forearms and palms may not come all the way together. Bring them as close as is comfortable.

Benefits: Range of motion in shoulders and arms, chest and upper back stretch, lymphatic drainage in arms

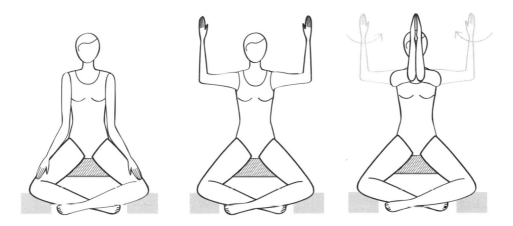

What is a yoga "chest opener"?

A chest opener (also sometimes called a "heart opener") is a common yoga term used to describe poses that stretch the muscles across the front of the chest and expand the front of the rib cage. This happens in coordination with the shoulders moving back as the shoulder blades draw toward each other. For many reasons, such as shoulder tension, poor posture, and stress, the chest often becomes compressed, therefore limiting full, free breathing. Among other benefits, chest opening can increase breathing capacity and support a positive shift in mood.

CACTUS TWIST

Sit upright with palms on your thighs.

INHALE: Lift arms to Cactus.

EXHALE: Holding your right Cactus arm steady, bring your left Cactus arm across to your right, twisting your spine to the right. Your forearms may or may not touch.

INHALE: Reopen your arms to Cactus.

EXHALE: Repeat on the second side, holding your left Cactus arm steady and twisting to the left as you bring your right forearm toward your left.

INHALE: Reopen to Cactus.

EXHALE: Lower palms to thighs.

Repeat the entire sequence three times.

Benefits: Range of motion in shoulders and arms, upper spine flexibility, chest and upper back stretch/strengthening, lymphatic drainage in upper body

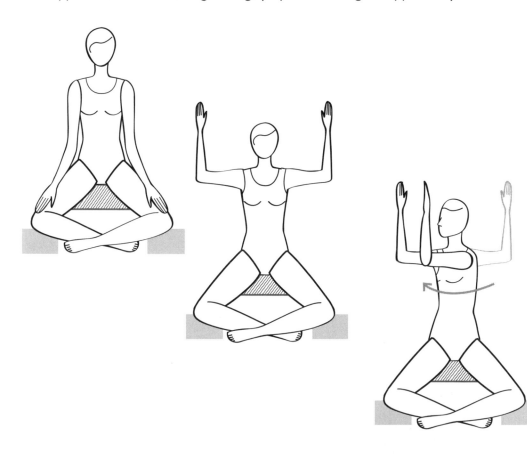

CACTUS TEAPOT

INHALE: Open arms to Cactus.

EXHALE: Lower your right hand to the floor or a block beside your right hip.

INHALE: Place your left hand behind your head and point your left elbow up like the handle of a teapot.

EXHALE: Lean farther to the right, as if pouring tea from your right shoulder.

Hold for three breaths before coming back upright. With each inhale find more length from your left hip to your left elbow. With each exhale lean slightly further to the right.

Repeat sequence on the opposite side, leaning to the left.

Benefits: Range of motion in shoulders and arms, upper spine flexibility, chest and upper back stretch/strengthening, lymphatic drainage in upper body

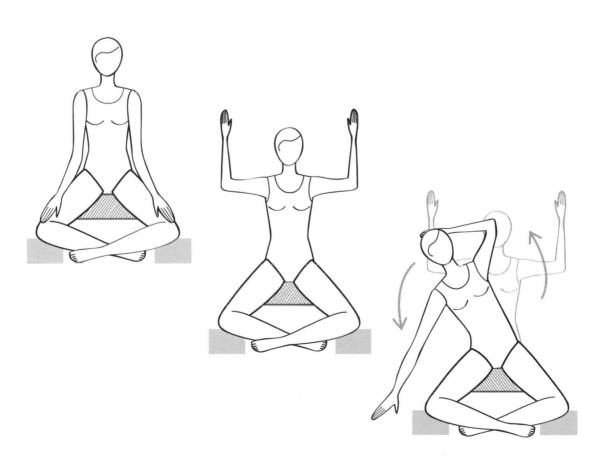

DIRTY T-SHIRT

INHALE: Lift arms to Cactus.

EXHALE: Fold left arm over right, giving yourself a hug.

INHALE: Begin to lift your elbows higher. As if taking off a T-shirt, slide your fingers up your arms as you reach your arms toward the ceiling. Expand your chest.

EXHALE: Lower palms to thighs.

Repeat sequence, this time folding right arm over left to give yourself a hug. Then repeat the entire sequence six times, alternating which arm is on top.

Modifications: The action of removing the imaginary T-shirt may be difficult if you are recovering from surgery. Modify by skipping this movement and returning to Cactus arms instead.

Benefits: Range of motion in shoulders and arms, chest and upper back stretch/ strengthening, lymphatic drainage in arms

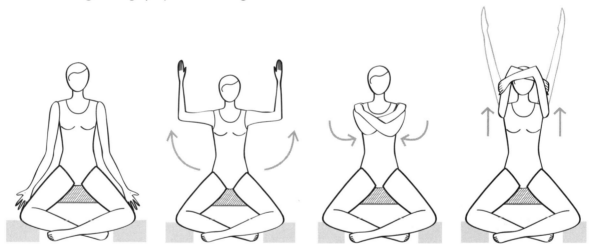

Why switch legs in a cross-legged seat?

When you sit in a cross-legged seat, you will notice you habitually place the same leg in front or on top. During seated practice such as warm-up arm vinyasas, if you are sitting cross-legged be sure to switch the crossing of your legs so that each leg gets equal time in each position. This will help to balance the flexibility and alignment of your hips.

SEATED CAT AND COW

Sit in a chair, cross-legged or in Hero pose. Cup your hands on your knees or thighs, extending your arms as much as possible.

INHALE: Arch your spine, lifting your chest up through your upper arms, belly moving toward your thighs. Keeping your legs firm and steady, pull your knees back with your hands to help draw your upper body forward.

EXHALE: Round your spine, belly away from thighs, head bowing forward, as if wrapping your torso over a beach ball. Press your hands against your knees.

Repeat sequence at least five times. If you are sitting cross-legged, switch which leg is on top after completing a few rounds so that you have done the sequence an equal number of times in each position.

Benefits: Full spine flexibility, chest and upper back stretch/strengthening, stimulates lymph system in hips and torso

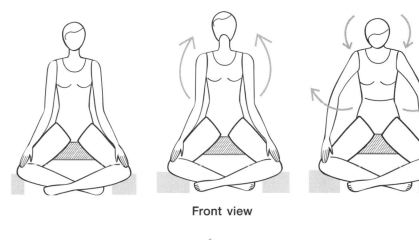

Front view

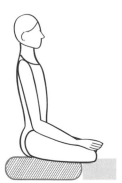
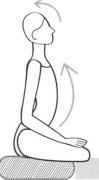
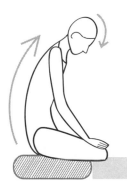

Side view

132

How to Build
Your Own
Yoga Practice

•

Seated Hip and
Spine Warm-Ups

KNEE-UP SEATED CAT AND COW

Sit cross-legged with your right leg in front. Place your right foot on the floor, your right knee pointing up, thigh close to your belly. Hold your right shin firmly with both hands.

INHALE: Arch your spine by moving your belly toward your thigh, broadening across your collarbones, lifting your heart and drawing your shoulder blades together.

EXHALE: Round your spine by drawing your belly away from your thigh and curling your head toward your knee.

Repeat five times. Then repeat sequence five times on the second side, holding your left leg.

Modifications: If your hips are tight it may be difficult to arch your spine. Try sitting on a higher support and bending your lifted knee a little less deeply so the foot that is on the floor is farther away from your hip.

Benefits: Hip stretch/mobility, spine flexibility, chest and upper back stretch/ strengthening, stimulates lymph system in hips and torso

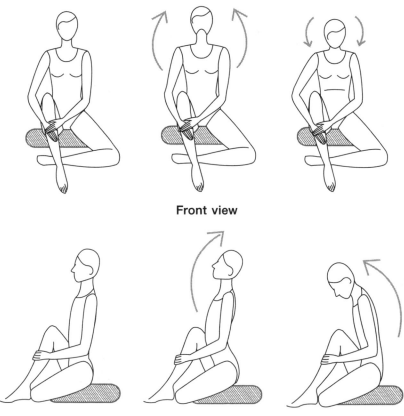

Front view

Side view

KNEE-UP SEATED TWIST

Begin from the same position as Knee-Up Seated Cat and Cow, with your right foot on the floor, knee bent.

INHALE: Sit fully upright, chest broad, crown of your head lifted.

EXHALE: Twist your belly and chest to the right. Place your left hand on your right shin and right hand to the floor or a block behind you. Turn your head to look past your right shoulder.

INHALE: Sit taller and slowly turn your head to look past your left shoulder.

EXHALE: Slowly turn your head back into the twist, gazing past your right shoulder.

Repeat five times. Then repeat the sequence five times on the second side, twisting to the left.

Modifications: If your hips are tight it may be difficult to sit upright. Try sitting on a higher support and bending your lifted knee a little less deeply so the foot that is on the floor is further away from your hip. If you experience any neck pain, do not turn your head as far into the twist.

Benefits: Hip stretch, spine flexibility, releases neck tension, stimulates lymph system in hips and torso

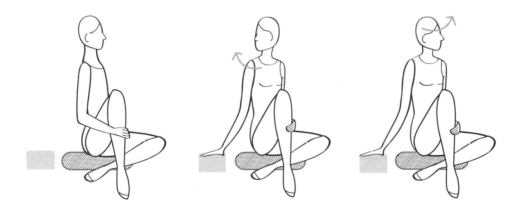

134

How to Build
Your Own
Yoga Practice

•

Warm-Ups
On Your Back—
Supine Vinyasas

Warm-Ups On Your Back—Supine Vinyasas

FULL-BODY STRETCH

Props needed: One bolster or two blankets

Lie on your back with your legs extended, arms by your sides, palms face down. Place the bolster or two folded blankets overhead (but not under your head).

Part 1

Start with both feet flexed (toes reaching back toward your head, heel pressing forward).

INHALE: Point your toes away from you.

EXHALE: Flex your feet, pulling your toes back toward you and reaching away with your heels.

Repeat three times.

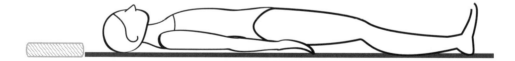

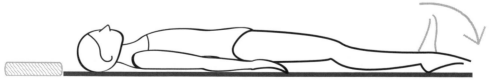

Part 1, pointing feet

135

Getting
Warmed Up

•

Warm-Ups
On Your Back—
Supine Vinyasas

FULL-BODY STRETCH

Part 2

Start with both feet flexed.

INHALE: Point toes while lifting both arms overhead until they rest on the bolster or blankets with palms face up.

EXHALE: Flex your feet while returning arms to your sides, palms down.

Repeat three times.

Modifications: If one or both arms do not reach the bolster overhead, add bolsters or blankets so that each arm can be fully supported. It is important to support both arms in a symmetrical way, despite any differences in mobility. Your less flexible side should determine the height of your support.

Benefits: Range of motion in shoulders and arms; strength/flexibility in feet, ankles, and legs; stimulates movement of lymph through the whole body; improves venous return from lower extremities

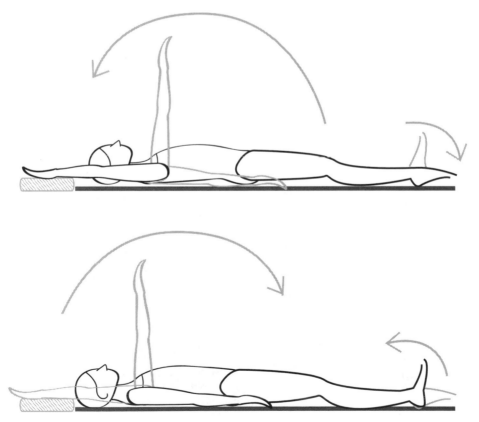

Part 2, pointing feet and lifting arms overhead

136

How to Build
Your Own
Yoga Practice

•

Warm-Ups
On Your Back—
Supine Vinyasas

LEG ROCKING

Lie on your back with knees bent, feet flat on the floor, knees and feet hip width apart.

Part 1

Lift and rotate your bent right leg so you can hold your right heel with your left hand. Flex your right foot. Support your right thigh or knee with your right hand. Draw your right shin toward your chest.

INHALE: Rock the lifted leg to the right.

EXHALE: Rock the lifted leg to the left. Keep your left leg stable, with the knee still bent, foot to the floor.

Repeat five times, coordinating the movement with your breath.

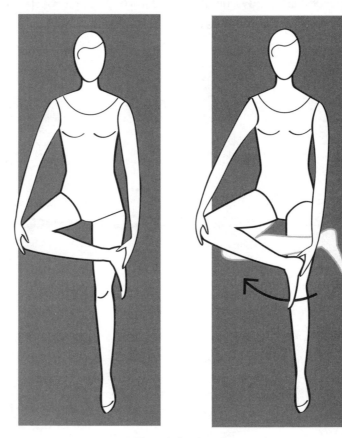

Part 1, legs only

LEG ROCKING

Part 2

INHALE: As you rock your leg to the right, turn your head to the left. Keep your head resting on the mat. Avoid tensing your neck.

EXHALE: As you rock your leg to the left, turn your head to the right.

Repeat five times. Then repeat part 1 and part 2 on the second side, lifting your left leg.

Modifications: For a gentler hip stretch, instead of drawing your shin toward your chest, rest your lifted ankle on the thigh of the opposite bent leg. Continue to rock your lifted leg with both hands, but allow your bottom leg to rock with it, assisting and supporting this movement.

Benefits: Hip stretch, hip joint mobility, releases neck tension

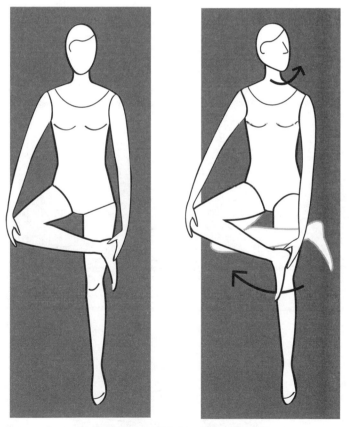

Part 2, with head turns

138

How to Build
Your Own
Yoga Practice

•

Warm-Ups
On Your Back—
Supine Vinyasas

CRUNCH AND SWITCH

Lie on your back with legs extended.

Part 1

Bend your left knee in toward your belly. Hold your left thigh with both hands.

INHALE: Point your right foot away from you while pulling your left knee closer to your belly.

EXHALE: Switch legs, pulling your right knee in and extending your left leg on the floor as you point your left foot away from you.

Repeat, switching legs six times.

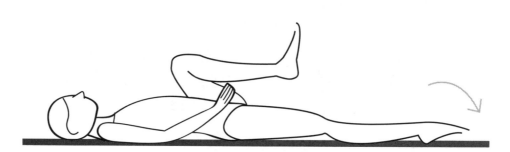

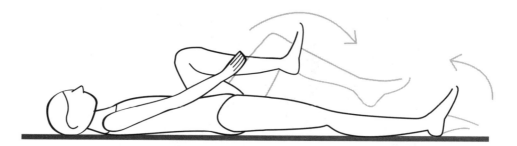

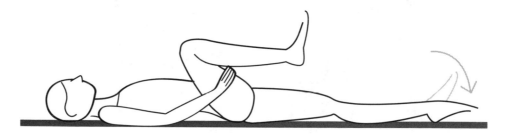

Part 1, legs only

139

Getting
Warmed Up
•
Warm-Ups
On Your Back—
Supine Vinyasas

CRUNCH AND SWITCH

Part 2

INHALE: Extend your right leg, pointing your right foot away from you while pulling your left knee toward you.

EXHALE: Gently lift your head toward the bent left knee.

INHALE: Rest your head back on the floor as you pull your right knee toward you and extend your left leg, pointing your left foot.

EXHALE: Gently lift your head toward the bent right knee.

Repeat, switching legs six times.

Benefits: Core strength, hip mobility; stimulates lymph system, especially in legs, hips, and abdomen; improves venous return from lower extremities

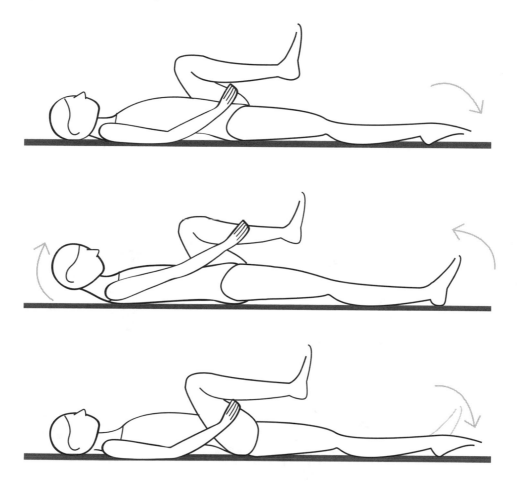

Part 2, with head lifts

140

How to Build
Your Own
Yoga Practice
•
Warm-Ups
On Your Back—
Supine Vinyasas

CRUNCH TWIST

Lie on your back. Bend both knees, pulling your thighs toward your belly with both hands. Lift your shins parallel to the floor so your body is in a chair shape. Squeeze your legs toward one another.

INHALE: Extend arms out to the sides, resting them on the floor at shoulder height with palms down.

EXHALE: Lean your chair legs to the left, without bringing them to the floor.

INHALE: Bring your chair legs back to center, above your hips.

EXHALE: Lean your chair legs to the right.

Repeat sequence twice. Then rest your feet on the floor and relax your abdominals, breathing naturally.

Modifications: To reduce the intensity of this sequence, move your chair legs only slightly to each side. To increase intensity, lower your chair legs so they hover just above the floor with each exhale.

Benefits: Core strength, hip strength and mobility, lower spine flexibility, lymphatic drainage from legs, improves venous return from lower extremities

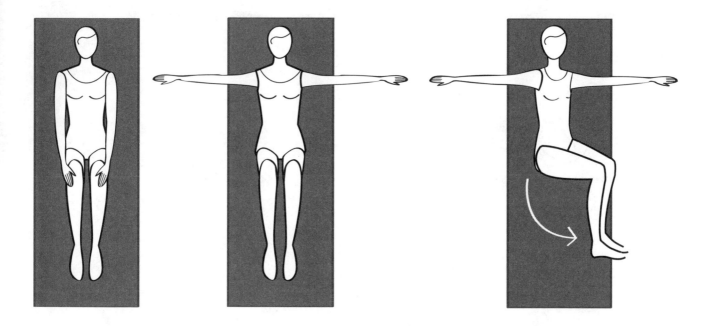

141

Getting
Warmed Up
•
Warm-Ups
On Your Back—
Supine Vinyasas

KNOCK-KNEED CACTUS

Props needed: Two folded blankets

Lie on your back with a folded blanket on either side of your shoulders. Open your arms to a cactus shape so the backs of your hands and forearms are resting on the blankets. Bend your knees, placing your feet as wide as the mat. Rest your knees against each other.

Part 1—Knock-Kneed Cactus Clap

INHALE: Broaden your chest with arms open in the cactus shape.

EXHALE: Bring your Cactus arms together in front of your face, trying to connect palms, forearms, and elbows.

INHALE: Open your Cactus arms out to rest on the blankets, broadening your chest.

EXHALE: Bring your cactus arms together.

Repeat three times.

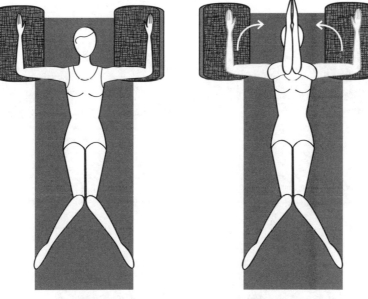

Part 1, Cactus Clap

142

How to Build
Your Own
Yoga Practice

•

Warm-Ups
On Your Back—
Supine Vinyasas

KNOCK-KNEED CACTUS

Part 2—Knock-Kneed Cactus Twist

INHALE: Begin in knock-kneed position with your Cactus arms resting on the blankets.

EXHALE: Bring your left Cactus arm across toward your right arm, keeping your right arm on the blanket. Let your head and upper spine follow your left arm as it pulls you into the twist, but keep both hips firmly on the floor.

INHALE: Bring your left arm back to the blanket opening into Cactus arms, broadening your chest.

Repeat three times. Then repeat three times on the second side, bringing your right arm toward your left.

Modifications: Depending on the shape of your legs or the tightness in your hips, your knees may not touch in the knock-kneed position. Allow your thighs to rest against each other instead. Limited mobility in your shoulders or chest may require additional blankets under your Cactus arms. As always, support both arms at the same height to maintain body symmetry. In both part 1 and part 2 your cactus arms may or may not touch on the exhale.

Benefits: Core strength, upper spine flexibility, chest opening, shoulder mobility, upper back stretch, releases tension in lower back

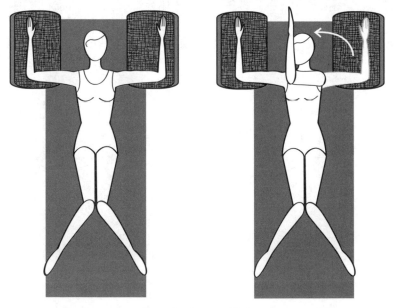

Part 2, Cactus Twist

143

Getting
Warmed Up
•
Warm-Ups
On Your Back—
Supine Vinyasas

How can I support my arms in a cactus shape?

Lying on your back with arms in a cactus shape, like in Knock-Kneed Cactus Twist and many of the restorative poses, often requires extra attention to support your arms in a comfortable position. In Cactus the elbow, forearm, wrist, and back of the hand should all be supported by the folded blanket. Often shoulder tightness causes the wrist and hand to be higher above the floor than the elbow, requiring additional support. If this is the case, fold a second blanket and place it under your wrist and hand, so that the props under each arm make the shape of a triangular wedge (lower at the elbow, higher at the hand) rather than a flat surface.

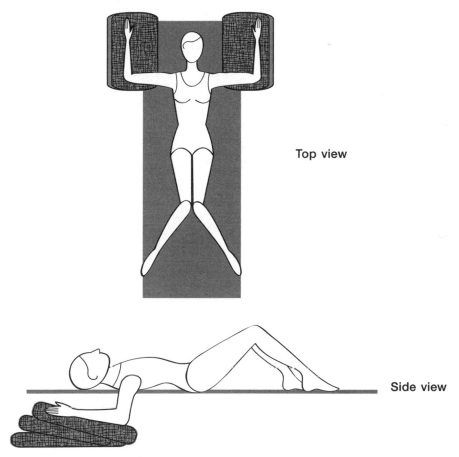

Top view

Side view

Supporting your arms in Cactus

144

How to Build
Your Own
Yoga Practice

•

Warm-Ups
on Hands
and Knees

Warm-Ups on Hands and Knees

HANDS AND KNEES POSITION

Place your hands directly under your shoulders, separating your fingers and feeling your entire palms connected to the floor. Place your knees slightly apart, under your hips. If your knees are uncomfortable on the floor, place a folded blanket under both knees. Rest the tops of your feet (toenail side down) on the floor. Find a neutral spine position, neither sagging your belly toward the floor nor rounding your back toward the ceiling, but keeping a flat back like a table. Your neck and head position are a continuation of your neutral spine. Reach the crown of your head forward, keeping your gaze on the floor.

How can I protect my wrists?

Particularly during hands-and-knees poses, if it is painful for you to put weight on your hands or wrists, or for any other reason you are concerned about weight bearing on your arms (for instance because of lymphedema), there is an alternative. Instead of placing your hands under your shoulders, you can support yourself on your forearms. In order to set this up properly you will need four blocks. Line up your blocks like parallel railroad tracks, with two blocks end-to-end on the left and two blocks end-to-end on the right, all blocks on the lowest level. The distance between the "railroad tracks" should be the width of your shoulders. Support your elbows, forearms, and palms on the two parallel lines of blocks, with elbows directly under your shoulders, so your forearms are now parallel to each other.

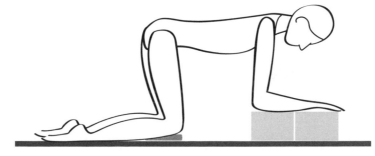

Modification to protect your wrists in hands and knees poses

145

Getting
Warmed Up
•
Warm-Ups
on Hands
and Knees

CAT AND COW

INHALE: Arch your spine by lifting your tail toward the ceiling and dipping your belly toward the floor. Broaden your chest, reaching it forward through your upper arms. Extend the crown of your head forward and slightly up, keeping the back of your neck long. Imagine you are a sway-backed cow.

EXHALE: Press your hands and shins into the floor and round your spine by curling your tailbone down and lifting the middle of your back toward the ceiling. Drop your head toward the floor, relaxing your neck completely. Imagine you're a spooked Halloween cat.

Repeat for ten breaths.

Modifications: If you feel tightness or a painful twinge in your back, make these movements even slower and more subtle, arching and rounding your spine to the degree you can without causing discomfort. Over time your spine will become more flexible.

Benefits: Spine and hip mobility; arm strengthening; stimulates lymph system in arms and torso; releases tension in lower back, upper back, and neck

146

How to Build
Your Own
Yoga Practice

•

Warm-Ups
on Hands
and Knees

HANDS AND KNEES TWIST

Part 1

Look down at your left hand.

INHALE: Reach your left arm straight out to the side at shoulder height, like an airplane wing, palm facing down. Follow your left hand with your eyes. Feel your shoulder blades actively drawing toward each other on your back. Keep your supporting right arm straight and strong.

EXHALE: Return your left hand to the floor under your shoulder. Follow the hand with your gaze.

Repeat three times. Then repeat three times on the right side, lifting your right arm.

Part 2

Look down at your left hand.

INHALE: Reach your left arm straight out to the side, turning your chest to the left to carry your arm a little higher toward the ceiling, creating a spinal twist and deeper chest opening. Follow your hand with your eyes.

EXHALE: Return your left hand to the floor under your shoulder.

Repeat three times. Then repeat three times on the right side.

Modifications: If the wrist of the supporting hand feels strained, try spreading your fingers wider and pressing them into the floor. If you are experiencing discomfort due to chest or abdominal surgery, try the Modified Hands and Knees Twist variation.

Benefits: Core strength, shoulder and arm strength/mobility, upper back strength/flexibility, stimulates lymph system in torso and arms, releases tension in upper back and neck

HANDS AND KNEES TWIST

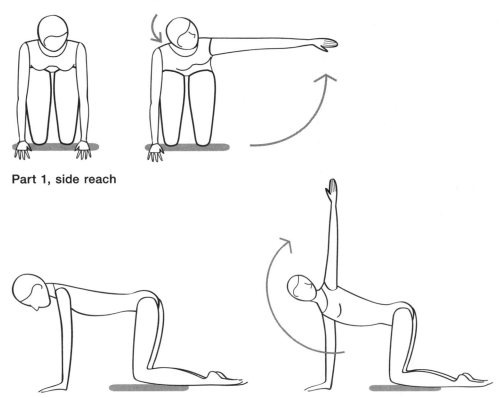

Part 1, side reach

Part 2, full twist

Modified Hands and Knees Twist

INHALE: Reach your left arm straight out to the side at shoulder height.

EXHALE: Bend your left elbow and tuck your hand behind your head. Cradle the back of your skull in the palm of your hand.

INHALE: Lift your left elbow a little higher, turning your chest to the left, shoulder blades drawing together on your back. Look to the left, letting the weight of your head rest in your palm.

EXHALE: Hang your left elbow toward the floor. Draw your abdominal muscles up toward your spine. Look back at your knees.

Repeat three times on each side.

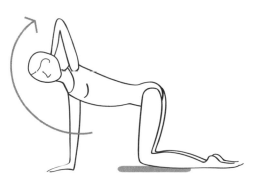

Arm modification

148

How to Build
Your Own
Yoga Practice

•

Warm-Ups
on Hands
and Knees

HANDS AND KNEES LEG EXTENSION

Part 1

INHALE: Extend your right leg back, toes tucked so the ball of your foot is on the floor, heel lifted.

Hold for three breaths. With each inhale reach your right heel and the crown of your head in opposite directions, actively lengthening your spine. With each exhale draw your abdominal muscles toward your spine, finding core support. At the end of the third breath:

EXHALE: Return to hands and knees position with your right knee under your hip.

Repeat on the second side, extending your left leg back.

Part 2

INHALE: Extend your right leg back, toes tucked on the floor.

EXHALE: Pull your right knee toward your nose, rounding your back into Cat pose. Lift your belly toward your spine. Hover your right foot above the floor.

INHALE: Extend your right leg back, toes tucked on the floor. Reach the crown of your head forward.

EXHALE: Return to hands and knees with a neutral spine.

Repeat three times on each side.

Modifications: If the wrist of the supporting hand feels strained, try spreading your fingers wider and pressing them into the floor. Also see the Modified Twist Extension variation on pages 152–53.

Benefits: Core strength, calf stretch, foot stretch, hip mobility, arm strengthening, stimulates the lymph system throughout the whole body

HANDS AND KNEES LEG EXTENSION

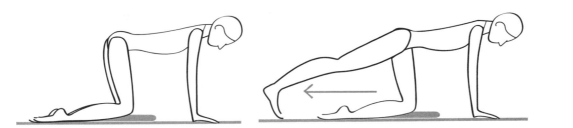

Part 1, leg extension

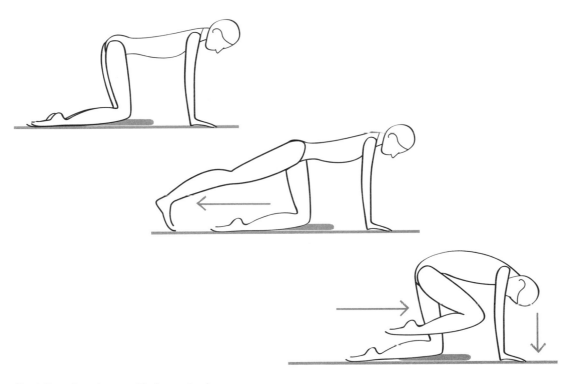

Part 2, extensions with knee tucks

150

How to Build
Your Own
Yoga Practice

•

Warm-Ups
on Hands
and Knees

TWIST EXTENSION

INHALE: Extend your right leg back, toes tucked on the floor.

EXHALE: Turn your right heel to the floor, pivoting your right foot to point away from you. Root the entire sole of the foot into the floor.

INHALE: Reach your right arm up toward the ceiling, turning your chest to the right. Take your gaze up and keep it on your right hand. Do not let your arm or hand fall behind your torso. Create an imaginary straight line between your left hand, shoulder blades, and right hand.

EXHALE: Release the breath by drawing your abdominal muscles inward toward the front of your spine.

INHALE: Lengthen again, reaching your right hand and arm up and press the left hand firmly into the floor.

EXHALE: Release the breath.

Lengthen and release with your arm lifted for three breaths.

Lower the arm and knee on an exhale, returning to hands and knees.

Repeat the entire sequence on the left side.

Modifications: If you find it difficult to balance in this position once you have reached your right leg back, pivot your bent left knee so your left foot points back behind you, creating a kickstand effect for greater stability.

Benefits: Core strength, chest opening, shoulder and arm strength/mobility, upper back strength, lymphatic drainage in arms, releases tension in upper back and neck

See pages 152–53 for Modified Twist Extension.

TWIST EXTENSION

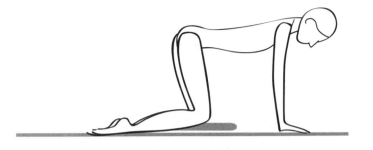

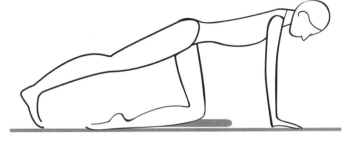

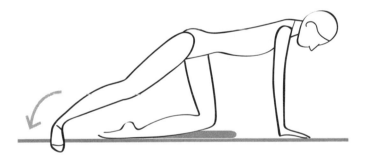

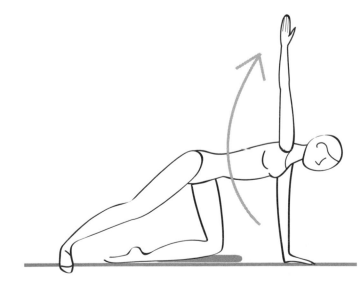

152

How to Build
Your Own
Yoga Practice

•

Warm-Ups
on Hands
and Knees

TWIST EXTENSION

Modified Twist Extension

INHALE: Extend your right leg back, toes tucked on the floor.

EXHALE: Turn your right heel to the floor, pivoting your right foot to point away from you. Root the entire sole of the foot into the floor.

INHALE: Reach your right arm straight out to the side at shoulder height.

EXHALE: Bend your right elbow and tuck your hand behind your head as you did for Modified Hands and Knees Twist (page 147).

INHALE: Lift your right elbow to point toward the ceiling. Turn your chest to the right in order to lift the elbow. Open your chest.

EXHALE: Hang your right elbow toward the floor. Draw your abdominal muscles up toward your spine. Relax your neck.

Lift and lower your elbow three times, following your breath.

Return to hands and knees position and repeat on the second side, extending your left leg back.

TWIST EXTENSION

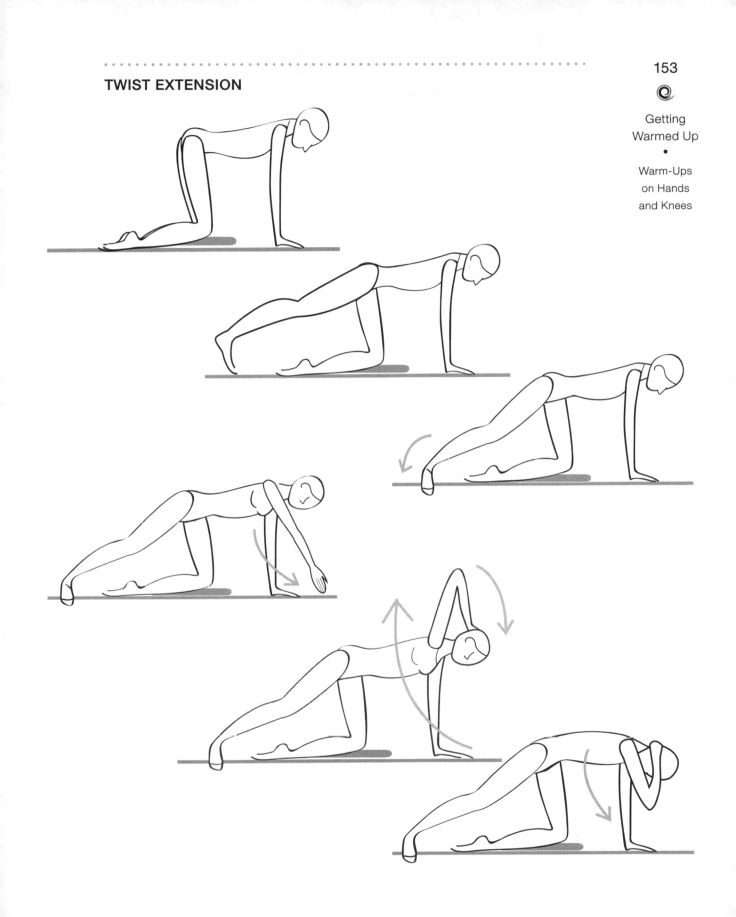

Belly-Down Poses—Prone Vinyasas

Lying belly-down is called the prone position. The word *prone* also means "to have a tendency or inclination." My favorite sleeping position is on my belly, so I am prone to sleeping prone. However I find many of the belly-down yoga poses challenging. The prone poses described here are modified to offer all the physical benefits of being belly-down, while avoiding potential discomfort and risk associated with specific cancers or surgeries.

Belly-down movement has special benefits for individuals who have had abdominal or gynecological surgeries. Surgery in the abdominal region can leave behind scar tissue or cause chronic lower back pain, vaginal prolapse, or pelvic organ prolapse related to bladder, colon, and prostate cancers. If ligaments that provide structural support to the pelvis have been removed, this can cause the pelvic bones to shift, the hips to widen, and the lower spine to become compressed. Certain surgeries can cause reduced blood flow in the pelvis, which may affect circulation in the legs and feet, potentially leading to neuropathy. Some cancer survivors suffer a loss of sensation in the abdomen, a diminished waistline, and bulging belly, in addition to lower back pain due to other cancer treatments.

Prone vinyasas stimulate the abdomen, increasing the circulation of blood and lymph. They massage and stretch abdominal muscles and scar tissue that are hard to access, while strengthening lower back muscles, therefore stabilizing and mobilizing both the front and the back of the spine. Pain reduction and better postural support can be the result.

The prone poses described here have been carefully modified so as not to be contraindicated for individuals recovering from abdominal, gynecological, and breast cancer surgeries, or breast reconstructions. The poses are practiced using a bolster or stack of folded blankets to support the thighs and hips in such a way that your belly, ribs, and breasts never touch the floor. This eliminates any discomfort or fear of pressure on the belly or chest.

. . . .

PRONE POSITION

In order to support your thighs and hips properly for these poses, lie belly-down across the bolster (or two folded blankets) so that your uppermost thighs and the front of both hips are supported, and your belly and lower thighs are suspended above the floor. Place your forearms on the floor, elbows under your shoulders, to support your upper body. Let the tops of your feet rest on the ground. If this causes discomfort in your foot or ankle, place a small rolled-up blanket under both ankles to relieve pressure.

SLUMBER PARTY

Props needed: Bolster or two blankets

Part 1

INHALE: In supported prone position, elongate the front of your body by reaching your toes back, spreading them wide, and reaching your chest forward through your upper arms. Press your forearms into the floor, spreading your fingers.

EXHALE: Draw your navel up toward your spine, pressing your thighs gently into the bolster. This will engage your core and lengthen your lower back.

Repeat five times.

Part 2

INHALE: Lift your chin to look forward as you lengthen the front of your body by reaching your toes back and your chest through your upper arms.

EXHALE: Release your head down toward the floor, relaxing the back of your neck, as you draw your navel up toward your spine, thighs pressing into the bolster.

Repeat five times.

Benefits: Core strength, abdominal stretch, releases tension in neck, releases tension in lower back, stimulates circulatory and lymph system in pelvis and abdomen

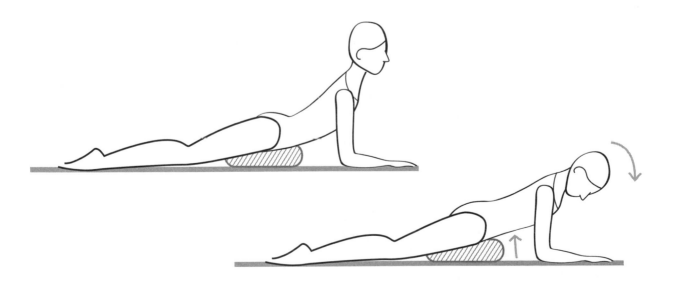

BUTT KICK (HALF BOW)

Props needed: Bolster or two blankets

Part 1

INHALE: In supported prone position, bend your left knee, kick your left heel toward your buttock. Lengthen your belly. Keep your chest lifted and open.

EXHALE: Lower the top of the left foot back to the mat. Relax your abdomen into the bolster.

Repeat five times with each leg.

Part 2

INHALE: Bend your left knee, bringing your foot toward your buttock.

EXHALE: Look over your right shoulder.

INHALE: Reach your left hand back toward the lifted foot and catch hold of your ankle if you can.

EXHALE: Holding your ankle, relax your thighs and hips into the bolster.

INHALE: Feel your belly lengthening. Keep your chest open.

EXHALE: Let the abdomen relax upward toward the spine.

Repeat the last inhale and exhale five times. Release your lifted foot and turn your head to center.

Repeat on the second side.

Modifications: In part 2, if you can't reach your foot, try looping a yoga strap or soft belt around your ankle and holding the strap instead. Or, instead of holding the ankle, continue the vinyasa by reaching for the ankle on each inhale, and then releasing your leg and arm back to the floor as you exhale.

Benefits: Abdominal, thigh, and hip stretch; spine flexibility; stimulates circulatory and lymph system in pelvis, abdomen, and legs

BUTT KICK (HALF BOW)

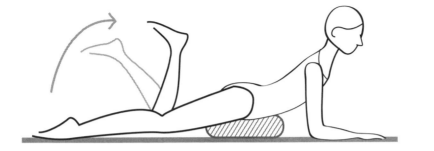

Part 1, warm-up kicks

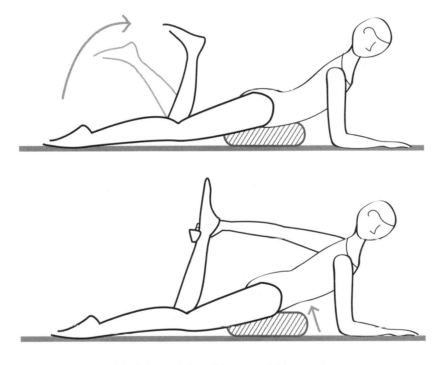

Part 2, with head turn and foot grab

158

How to Build
Your Own
Yoga Practice

•

Getting up
and Down

Getting Up and Down

Getting up and down from the floor with grace and ease is both a useful and empowering yoga tool. While it may not be a NASA shuttle launch, it can seem like a long way to go. Physical conditions such as stiffness, injury, or surgery can make it challenging and seemingly prohibitive to transition from standing to lying on the ground, or vice versa. However, by using proper body alignment, a few props, and a good measure of mindfulness, I have found that almost everyone who walks into my yoga class can learn to get safely up from and down to the floor. Here are two ways to conscientiously execute this transition as we move from warm-ups to standing and balancing poses.

TOE MASSAGE TO STAND

Props needed: Two blocks

Start in hands and knees position. Then place two blocks (on their highest level) on either side of your feet. Return your hands to the mat under your shoulders. Tuck your toes under, so the balls of your feet are on the floor.

Walk your hands back toward your knees as you shift your hips toward your heels. You may already begin to feel a toe stretch here. Lift your hands and place them on the blocks.

Pressing your hands into the blocks, rock your knees up away from the floor to perch on the balls of your feet, sitting on your heels. You can spend a few breaths here, rocking your weight gently forward and back on your feet for a toe massage.

To continue up to standing, press your feet into the floor and unfold your body like an accordion into an upright position.

Modifications: This series may not be appropriate if you have toe, foot, or knee pain or injury. You may want to try the Lunge to Stand sequence described below instead. If your flexibility allows, this sequence can also be done without the blocks.

Benefits: Increases circulation, flexibility, and sensation in toes and feet; builds confidence and mobility.

TOE MASSAGE TO STAND

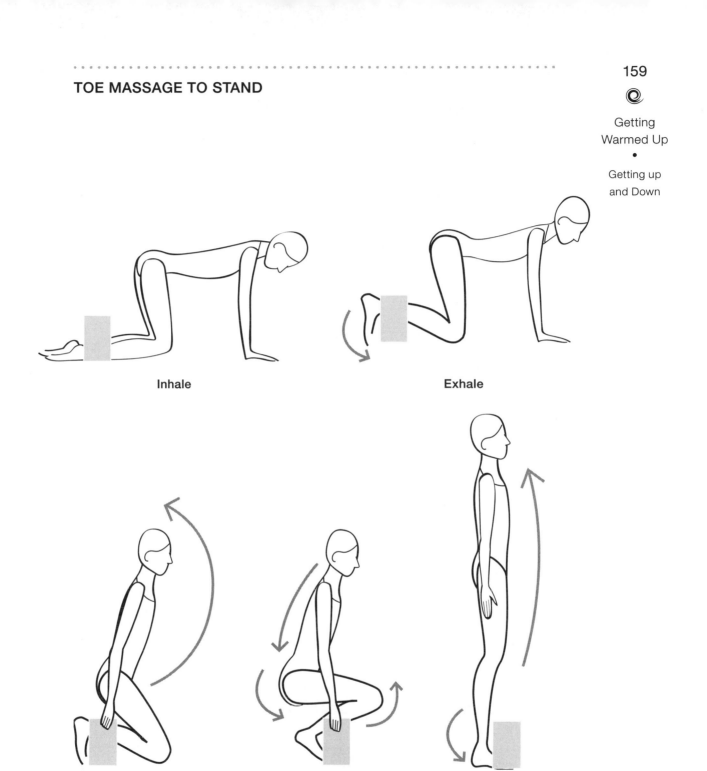

Inhale

Exhale

Inhale

Exhale
(rock forward and back
for a few breaths)

Inhale

160

How to Build
Your Own
Yoga Practice
•
Getting up
and Down

LUNGE TO STAND

Props needed: Two blocks

Starting in a hands and knees position with hands under your shoulders, place a block under each hand to raise your upper body. Step your left foot between the blocks, with the knee bent directly above the ankle. Tuck your right toes under so the ball of the foot is on the floor, and lift your right knee away from the ground.

Keeping your chest lifted, step your right foot forward between the blocks to join your left. Press both feet into the floor to straighten your legs, unfolding your body to stand fully upright.

Modifications: The block naturally has three height choices. I suggest starting with the highest and then experiment. When on the right height, the block creates space to bring your back foot forward with ease. This sequence can also be done without blocks depending on your flexibility and strength.

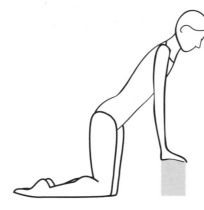

Inhale

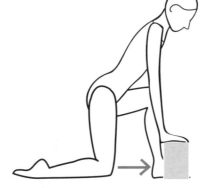

Exhale

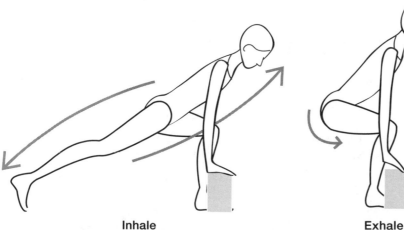

Inhale

Exhale

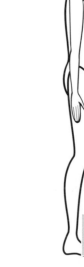

Inhale

BUILDING STRENGTH, BONES, AND BALANCE

Standing Poses

STAND TALL

Stand with feet hip width apart on your mat. Lift all your toes away from the floor without looking down at your feet. Feel your weight on the balls of your feet and your heels, your leg muscles active. Rock gently forward and back on your feet until you feel your weight is evenly balanced, front to back. Spread your toes apart from each other, and relax them back onto the floor.

Place your hands on your hips. Find a neutral position for your hips, in which you are neither rocking your hips forward nor tucking your tail under (see "Pelvic Tilt" on page 123). Press your hands down on your hips, feeling the rootedness of your legs and feet.

Place your hands on your side ribs. Lift your ribs up away from your hips, elongating your waist. Release your arms by your sides, maintaining the awareness in your feet, legs, hips, and rib cage that you have created. Relax your shoulders away from your ears.

Bring your chin parallel to the floor. Align your head directly above your pelvis and the soles of your feet. Imagine your feet reaching down into the earth like tree roots growing into the soil. Visualize your spine and the crown of your head extending upward like the trunk of the tree. Stand tall.

Benefits: Postural awareness; improves balance; activates muscles in feet, legs, and core; builds bone mass; spinal alignment to release tension in neck, shoulders, and back.

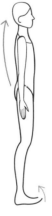
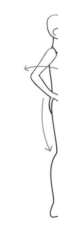
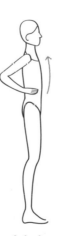
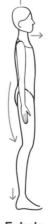

Inhale   Exhale   Inhale   Exhale

SWAY IN THE WIND (BEND LIKE A TREE)

INHALE: Stand tall.

EXHALE: Lean to the right, pouring weight into the right foot.

INHALE: Come back to the stand tall position with weight centered on the feet.

EXHALE: Lean to the left, pouring weight into the left foot.

INHALE: Stand tall.

EXHALE: As you lean to the right, lift your left arm out and up alongside your ear in a circular motion, palm facing in the direction you are leaning. Feel your left side stretch.

INHALE: Stand tall, releasing your left arm back by your side.

EXHALE: As you lean to the left, lift your right arm up into the side stretch.

Repeat three times to each side.

Modifications: If lifting the arm up beside the ear is difficult, for instance due to muscle tension, recent surgery, or scar tissue, lift the arm to the degree that is comfortable. You may also modify by bending the elbow of the lifted arm.

Benefits: Side body flexibility, shoulder and arm strength/mobility, improves balance, builds bone mass, lymphatic drainage in arms

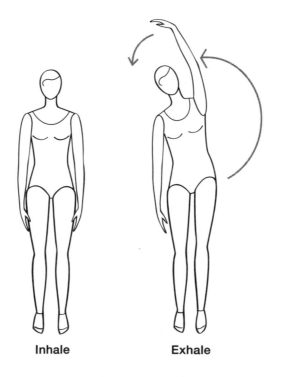

Inhale   **Exhale**

SWAN WINGS

Stand tall.

INHALE: Rotate your arms so the palms of your hands face forward and then out away from your body, thumbs pointing out and slightly back (see "Thumbs-Up" on page 126). Broaden your chest as your shoulder blades move toward each other.

EXHALE: Rotate your arms so your palms face in toward your thighs again.

INHALE: Begin by turning your palms to face out, then reach your arms out and up toward the ceiling in a circular motion to a comfortable position overhead with palms facing each other.

EXHALE: Lower your arms in a circular motion, like closing wings, until arms rest by your sides with palms facing your thighs, arriving back in the stand tall position.

Repeat for ten breaths, feeling your breath as the wind under your swan wings.

Modifications: If lifting your arms up high is difficult, for instance due to muscle tension, recent surgery, or scar tissue, raise your arms to your comfort level. Shoulder height is a fine place to stop as you work to lift your arms slightly higher with each repetition.

Benefits: Shoulder and arm strength/mobility, builds bone mass, lymphatic drainage in arms

Inhale   Exhale   Inhale   Exhale

CHAIR POSE

Stand tall. Place your hands on your hips, pointing your elbows slightly back.

INHALE: Open your chest.

EXHALE: Bend your knees as if beginning to sit in a chair. Engage your lower abdominal muscles and drop your tailbone.

INHALE: Place your hands on top of your thighs. Press your hands down as you expand your chest upward.

EXHALE: Bend your knees a little more deeply, continuing to lift and expand your chest. Keep the soles of your feet fully planted on the floor. Do not lift your toes or your heels.

Complete three breath cycles before returning to the stand tall position.

Modifications: If you feel pain in your knees, bend the knees less. If you wish to make this more challenging, bend your knees more deeply and sit lower. However, hips should never go below the level of the knees, and soles of the feet should stay planted on the floor.

Benefits: Leg, hip, and core strength; builds bone mass; improves balance; increases circulation

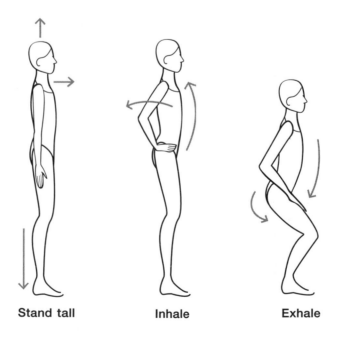

Stand tall   **Inhale**   **Exhale**

CRESCENT MOON

Stand tall.

INHALE: Reach your arms out and up like swan wings.

EXHALE: With arms lifted, turn your palms to face away from each other.

INHALE: Catch hold of your left wrist with your right hand and gently pull the arm upward.

EXHALE: Lean your upper body to the right, into a side bend. Continue to gently pull the left arm with the right hand. Keep both feet firmly planted on the floor and your chest facing forward.

INHALE: Come back upright, still holding your wrist.

EXHALE: Lean again to the right, into the side bend.

Repeat five times, following your breath. Then return to the stand tall position and switch to the second side, holding your right wrist with your left hand and side bending five times to the left.

Modifications: If it is challenging to lift your arms high, or to straighten the arms, lift your arms only as high as is comfortable and keep the elbows slightly bent.

Benefits: Side body flexibility, shoulder and arm strength/mobility, improves balance, builds bone mass, lymphatic drainage in arms

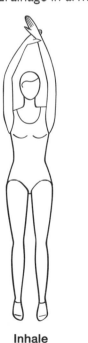

Inhale—reach arms out and up,   **Inhale**   **Exhale**
Exhale—turn palms out

DOWN DOG AT THE WALL

Props needed: Wall

Stand facing the wall with feet hip width apart and both arms extended, palms flat to the surface of the wall. Place your hands shoulder width apart, with middle fingers pointing straight up.

Begin to walk your feet away from the wall. As you do, bend forward at your hips to a ninety-degree angle and walk your hands down the wall until they are at the height of your hips. Align your body in an L-shape, with feet flat to the floor, palms flat to the wall. Keep your head lifted so your ears are between your upper arms.

INHALE: Bend your knees and elbows slightly. Lift your chest and look toward the wall.

EXHALE: Straighten your legs and arms, returning your head and neck to the original position. Press your palms actively into the wall, root your feet into the floor. Feel your lower belly engage, lifting up toward your spine.

Repeat five times, bending and straightening legs and arms with your breath.

Modifications: Tightness in your legs or hips may not allow you to fully straighten your legs in this pose. Modify with knees slightly bent throughout the sequence. If you feel too much stress in your shoulders or chest, try bringing your hands a little above hip height on the wall. Make sure you are not dropping your head toward the floor, which puts more stress on the shoulders.

Benefits: Full body stretch and strengthening; improves flexibility in legs, hips, spine, belly, chest, sides, shoulders, and arms; strengthens core, legs, shoulders, and arms; builds bone mass

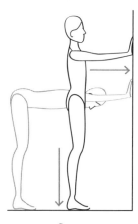
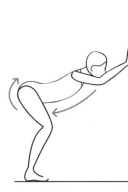
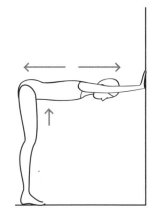

Start   **Inhale**   **Exhale**

Sun Salutations

The Sun Salutation, a traditional sequence of poses, is presented here in the y4c method, which offers the benefits of the classic version while avoiding positions and poses that may be harmful for cancer patients and survivors. Deep forward bends are avoided due to the increased risk of osteoporosis during and after chemotherapy treatment, since bones in the spine that are compressed during forward bends are the most common to weaken and break. Downward Dog and Plank poses are avoided, as full weight bearing on the arms is often contra-indicated by oncologists due to risks relating to surgery or lymphedema. The y4c method specially tailors the Sun Salutations using props to encourage enhanced chest opening in order to counteract any tendency to collapse the shoulders, chest, and belly due to surgery, fatigue, or depression. Keeping your chest wide and lifted throughout these sequences activates core strength that will support your spine in more challenging poses. Even experienced yogins can benefit from practicing this sequence, using props to enhance awareness of the abdominal muscles and deepen breathing.

**Why is it important to keep
my bent knee above my ankle?**

During Sun Salutation lunges, Warrior poses, and Side Angle, it is impor-tant to keep the bent knee directly above the ankle. Bending the knee past the ankle in weight-bearing poses such as lunges and Warrior poses causes instability in the knee joint and can potentially lead to injury. Keeping your knee above your ankle helps you to properly engage your leg muscles and evenly distribute weight along the bottom of your foot from heel to toe, improving balance and stabilizing the alignment of your whole body in the pose. If it is too strenuous to bend your knee over your ankle, bring your two feet closer together in these poses so that less bending is needed to achieve this alignment. (See "How far apart should my feet be in standing poses?" on page 178.)

STEP BACK SUN SALUTATION

Props needed: Two blocks

Place two blocks shoulder width apart on the highest level at the front of your mat. Stand tall between them. Line up your toes with the front edge of the blocks.

Part 1

INHALE: Reach your arms out and up like swan wings.

EXHALE: Bend your knees as if you're going into Chair pose and lower your arms, bringing your hands to the blocks.

INHALE: Straighten your legs, reaching arms out and up like swan wings.

EXHALE: Return your arms to your sides.

Repeat three times.

Part 2

INHALE: Reach your arms out and up like swan wings.

EXHALE: Bend your knees as if you're going into Chair pose and lower your arms, placing your hands on the blocks.

INHALE: Step your right leg back into a lunge. Reach the crown of your head forward while reaching back through your right heel. Your left knee should be directly above your left ankle.

EXHALE: Step your right foot forward again into Chair pose with your hands on the blocks, chest lifted.

INHALE: Straighten your legs, reaching arms out and up like swan wings.

EXHALE: Lower your arms to stand tall position.

Repeat on the second side, stepping your left foot back.

Modifications: If range of motion in your arms is limited, lift your arms only to a comfortable height. If your hands do not reach the blocks as you bend your knees from a standing position, stack two blocks under each hand.

Benefits: Strengthens the whole body, improves balance, builds bone mass, stimulates the lymph system, lymphatic drainage in arms, increases heart rate for cardiovascular health

STEP BACK SUN SALUTATION

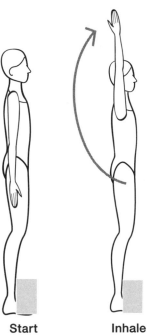
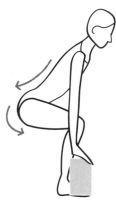

Start　　**Inhale**　　**Exhale**

Part 1, preparation

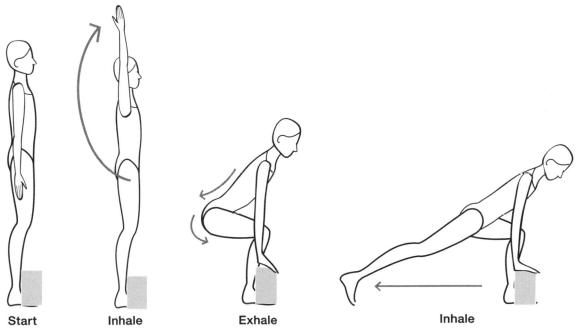

Start　　**Inhale**　　**Exhale**　　**Inhale**

Part 2, add step back

KNEE-DOWN SUN SALUTATION

Props needed: Two blocks, blanket (optional)

Place two blocks shoulder width apart on the highest level at the front of your mat. Stand tall between them. Line up your toes with the front edge of the blocks.

INHALE: Reach your arms out and up like swan wings.

EXHALE: Bend your knees as if you're going into Chair pose and bring your hands onto the blocks. Keep your chest lifted.

INHALE: Step your right leg back into a lunge. Reach the crown of your head forward while reaching back through your right heel. Left knee should be directly above left ankle.

EXHALE: Lower your right knee to the mat or a blanket, untucking your toes so the top of the foot rests on the floor.

INHALE: Lift your arms out and up, bringing your torso upright.

To complete the Sun Salutation, repeat each of these actions in reverse, following the illustrations from right to left.

EXHALE: Lower hands to blocks.

INHALE: Tuck right toes under and lift your right knee.

EXHALE: Step your right foot forward between the blocks, both knees bent, chest lifted.

INHALE: Straighten your legs, reaching your arms out and up like swan wings.

EXHALE: Lower your arms. Return to stand tall position.

Repeat on the second side, stepping back with your left leg.

Modifications: For sensitive knees, set a folded blanket across the middle of your mat where your knees will land during the knee-down lunge. If range of motion in your arms is limited, lift your arms only to a comfortable height. If your hands do not reach the blocks as you bend your knees from a standing position, stack two blocks under each hand.

Benefits: Strengthens the whole body, improves balance, builds bone mass, stimulates the lymph system, lymphatic drainage in arms, increases heart rate for cardiovascular health

KNEE-DOWN SUN SALUTATION

Start **Inhale** **Exhale** **Inhale**

Exhale **Inhale**

What does it mean to "lift my chest"?

In Sun Salutations you'll move through Chair pose, stepping back into a lunge as you keep your chest lifted. Keeping the chest liftted means that your chest remains above the level of your hips. It also means that your chest remains open (see "What is a yoga 'chest opener'?" on page 127) and actively reaching upward, as if there were a string connected to the center of your chest attached to a helium balloon. With this intention, even as you bend your knees and lower your hips, your chest continues to lift and expand.

STEP BACK TWIST

Props needed: Two blocks, blanket (optional)

Place two blocks shoulder width apart on the highest level at the front of your mat. Stand tall between them. Line up your toes with the front edge of the blocks.

INHALE: Reach your arms out and up like swan wings.

EXHALE: Bend your knees as if you're going into Chair pose and bring your hands onto the blocks. Keep your chest lifted.

INHALE: Step your left leg back into a lunge. Reach the crown of your head forward while reaching back through your left heel. Right knee should be directly above right ankle.

EXHALE: Lower your left knee to the mat or a blanket, untucking your toes so the top of the foot rests on the floor.

INHALE: Reach your right arm out and up toward the ceiling, turning your chest to the right as you did for Hands and Knees Twist (page 146). Follow your right hand with your gaze.

EXHALE: Lower your right hand back onto the block.

Repeat this twist to the right three times, following your breath.

Once both hands are back on the blocks:

INHALE: Tuck left toes under and lift your left knee into a lunge.

EXHALE: Step your left foot forward between the blocks, both knees bent, chest lifted.

INHALE: Straighten your legs, reaching your arms out and up like swan wings.

EXHALE: Lower your arms. Return to stand tall position.

Repeat on the second side, stepping back with your right leg and twisting to the left.

Modifications: For sensitive knees, set a folded blanket across the middle of your mat where your knees will land during the knee-down lunge.

Benefits: Spine flexibility, strengthens the whole body, improves balance, builds bone mass, stimulates the lymph system, lymphatic drainage in arms, increases heart rate for cardiovascular health

STEP BACK TWIST

Modified Step Back Twist

A modified version of Step Back Twist that's similar to Modified Hands and Knees Twist (see page 147) can be applied once you have reached the twisting part of the Sun Salutation.

INHALE: Reach your right arm straight out to the side at shoulder height.

EXHALE: Bend your right elbow and tuck your hand behind your head. Cradle the back of your skull in the palm of your hand.

INHALE: Lift your right elbow a little higher, turning your chest to the right, shoulder blades drawing together on your back. Look to the right.

EXHALE: Hang your right elbow toward the block on which your right hand had been resting. Draw your abdominal muscles up toward your spine.

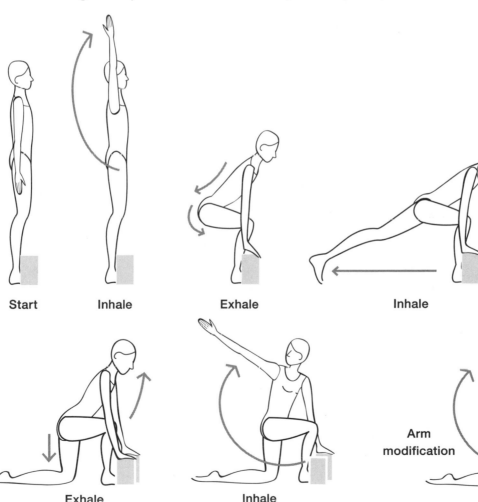

Start   Inhale   Exhale   Inhale

Exhale   Inhale   Arm modification

STEP BACK SEESAW

Place two blocks shoulder width apart on the highest level at the front of your mat. Stand tall between them. Line up your toes with the front edge of the blocks.

INHALE: Reach your arms out and up like swan wings.

EXHALE: Bend your knees as if going into Chair pose and bring your hands onto the blocks. Keep your chest lifted.

INHALE: Step your right leg back into a lunge. Reach the crown of your head forward while reaching back through your right heel. Left knee should be directly above left ankle.

EXHALE: Push your left foot into the floor to straighten your left leg. Keep your chest open and reaching forward.

INHALE: Bend your left knee over your left ankle.

Repeat the movement of bending and straightening your left leg five times, following your breath. To complete the Sun Salutation:

EXHALE: Step your right foot forward between the blocks, both knees bent, chest lifted.

INHALE: Straighten your legs, reaching your arms out and up like swan wings.

EXHALE: Lower your arms. Return to stand tall position.

Repeat on the second side, stepping your left leg back into a lunge, straightening and bending your right leg.

Modifications: Tight hamstrings may prevent you from fully straightening the front leg. Straighten only as much as you can without forcing into the stretch. If range of motion in your arms is limited, lift your arms only to a comfortable height. If your hands do not reach the blocks as you bend your knees from a standing position, stack two blocks under each hand.

Benefits: Hamstring flexibility, strengthens the whole body, improves balance, builds bone mass, stimulates the lymph system, increases heart rate for cardiovascular health

STEP BACK SEESAW

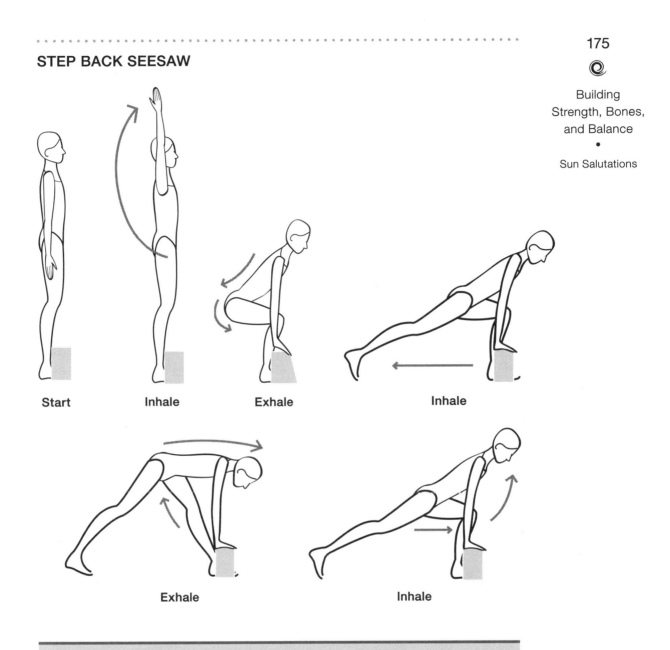

Start   **Inhale**   **Exhale**   **Inhale**

Exhale   **Inhale**

What does it mean to "follow my breath"?

Watching your breath, following your breath, and moving with your breath can sound deceptively simple. But just breathing consciously can be surprisingly challenging. The directive to follow your breath during a yoga movement sequence means that you are observing the natural length of your inhale and exhale and moving your body in coordination with your breathing. Your breath leads, setting the pace, and your body follows. This requires both precise, focused attention and letting go of control.

Warrior Poses

WARRIOR ONE

Props needed: Two blocks

Place two blocks shoulder width apart on the highest level at the front of your mat. Stand tall between them. Line up your toes with the front edge of the blocks.

INHALE: Reach your arms out and up like swan wings.

EXHALE: Bend your knees as if going into Chair pose and bring your hands onto the blocks. Keep your chest lifted.

INHALE: Step your right leg back into a lunge. Look forward while reaching back through your right heel. Left knee should be directly above left ankle.

EXHALE: Bring your right heel down to the mat, placing your foot at an angle so your toes point toward your right hand.

INHALE: Lift your torso to an upright position, placing both hands on your left thigh.

EXHALE: Draw your belly back toward your spine.

INHALE: If you feel steady and have the core support to stay balanced here, then reach your arms forward and up.

Hold Warrior One for three complete breaths.

EXHALE: Lower hands to blocks.

INHALE: Lift your right heel away from the floor and turn your foot so the toes face forward and heel points to the back of your mat.

EXHALE: Step your right foot forward between the blocks, both knees bent, chest lifted.

INHALE: Straighten your legs, reaching your arms out and up like swan wings.

EXHALE: Lower your arms. Return to stand tall position.

Repeat on the second side, stepping back with the left leg.

Modifications: If range of motion in your arms is limited, lift your arms only to a comfortable height. If your hands do not reach the blocks as you bend your knees from a standing position, stack two blocks under each hand.

Benefits: Strengthens the whole body, improves balance, builds bone mass, stimulates the lymph system, lymphatic drainage in arms, increases heart rate for cardiovascular health

WARRIOR ONE

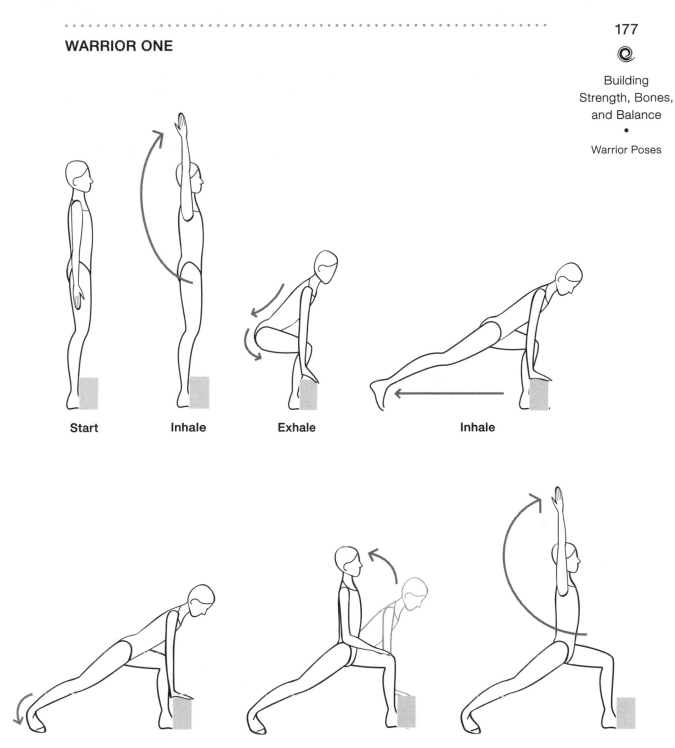

Start **Inhale** **Exhale** **Inhale**

Exhale **Inhale—torso upright,
Exhale—belly to spine** **Inhale**

WARRIOR TWO

Turn to face the long side of your mat. Separate your feet wide apart (or a comfortable, stable distance) with feet parallel. Reach your arms out to the sides at shoulder level, palms down.

Turn your left toes to face toward the short side of your mat. Keep your hips level. Your chest will remain facing the long side of your mat. Turn your head to gaze past your left fingertips.

Bend your left knee until it is over your left ankle.

Hold Warrior Two for three breaths. As you inhale, feel your chest broaden, arms reaching out in opposite directions. As you exhale, root your feet into the floor and engage your legs; move your lower belly in and up.

To release from the pose, straighten your left knee. Pivot your left foot in, parallel to your right. Repeat on the second side, turning out your right foot.

Modifications: The degree to which you separate your feet will depend on the flexibility, strength, and length of your legs. Modify as needed, making sure that whatever distance you choose, your bent knee does not go past the ankle.

Benefits: Hip mobility, leg strength/flexibility, arm and shoulder strength, core activation, improves balance, builds bone mass, stimulates lymph system, increases heart rate for cardiovascular health

How far apart should my feet be in standing poses?

As you make your way into Warrior Two or Triangle pose you begin by separating your feet wide apart. But how wide? The answer depends on your body—the length of your legs, your flexibility, your strength, your balance, and your comfort. Find a stance that allows you to feel stable but challenged. When you move into Warrior Two, as you bend one knee over your ankle notice whether your knee tends to go past the ankle. If so, lengthen your stance. If it is a struggle to bend the knee deep enough for ankle above knee alignment, shorten your stance. (See "Why is it important to keep my bent knee above my ankle?" on page 167.) Warrior Two is the basis for your alignment in Side Angle and Triangle pose, so once you have found your stance here you can apply it to the other poses.

WARRIOR TWO

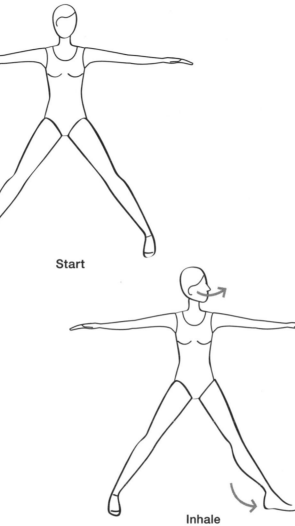

Start

Inhale

Exhale

SIDE ANGLE

Props needed: Two blocks

Begin in Warrior Two with your left knee bent and a block behind your left ankle on the highest level.

EXHALE: Lean to the left, placing your left hand on the block with your arm straight. Rest your right arm along your right side.

INHALE: Reach your right arm straight up toward the ceiling.

Hold Side Angle for three breaths. As you inhale, reach the crown of your head and your right foot in opposite directions, lengthening your whole body. As you exhale, root both feet into the floor with equal weight and turn your chest open toward the ceiling, gazing up toward your lifted arm.

To release from the pose, return to Warrior Two. Straighten your bent leg and bring your feet to parallel. Repeat on the second side, placing the block behind your right ankle.

Modifications: If it is difficult to reach the block with your bottom hand without feeling compressed in your hip or waist, stack two blocks under your hand for additional height. If tightness in the shoulder, chest, or arm makes it difficult to lift the upper arm toward the ceiling, lift only to a comfortable level, leave at your side, or modify by bending the elbow of the lifted arm and putting your hand behind your head. Also, like Warrior Two, the degree to which you separate your feet will depend on the flexibility, strength, and length of your legs. Modify as needed, making sure that whatever distance you choose, your bent knee does not go past the ankle.

Benefits: Hip mobility, leg strength/flexibility, arm and shoulder strength/mobility, side stretch, core activation, improves balance, builds bone mass, lymphatic drainage in arms, stimulates lymph system, increases heart rate for cardiovascular health

SIDE ANGLE

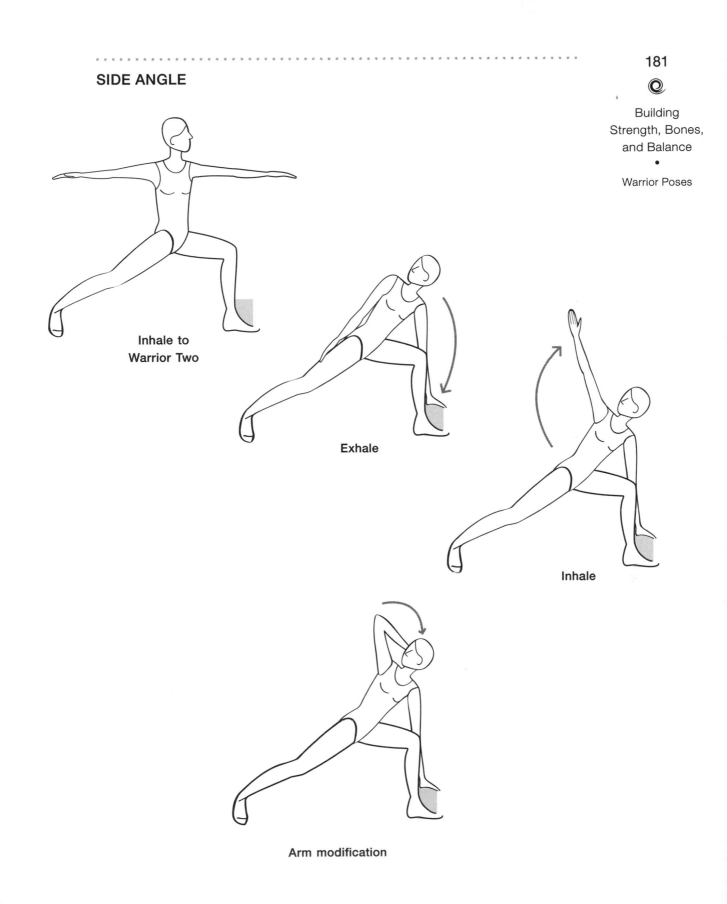

**Inhale to
Warrior Two**

Exhale

Inhale

Arm modification

TRIANGLE

Props needed: One block

Turn to face the long side of your mat. Separate your feet wide apart (or a comfortable, stable distance) with feet parallel. Place a yoga block on the highest level behind your left ankle.

Turn your left toes to face toward the short side of your mat. Keep your hips level. Your chest will remain facing the long side of your mat. Reach your arms out to the sides at shoulder level, palms down. Turn your head to gaze past your left fingertips.

Initiating the movement from your hips, tilt your upper body to the left, keeping both sides of your waist long. Place your left hand onto the block. Reach your right arm straight up, palm facing out in the same direction as your chest, hand directly above your shoulder. Maintain your upper body in the same plane as your lower body, as if you were pressed between two sheets of glass.

Hold Triangle for three breaths. As you inhale reach your arms in opposite directions, feeling your chest wide. As you exhale root both feet equally into the floor and turn your chest open toward the ceiling. Gaze up toward your lifted hand.

To release from the pose, tilt your spine upright. Bring your hands to your hips. Pivot your left foot in, parallel to your right. Repeat on the second side, placing the block behind your right ankle.

Modifications: If it is difficult to reach the block with your bottom hand while keeping the legs straight, stack two blocks under the hand for additional height. If tightness in the shoulder, chest, or arm makes it difficult to lift the upper arm toward the ceiling, lift only to a comfortable level, or rest the upper arm on your side like in leaning Side Angle (page 181). If gazing up toward the lifted hand strains your neck, instead look forward in the same direction as your chest. Also, like Warrior Two, the degree to which you separate your feet will depend on the flexibility, strength, and length of your legs. Modify as needed, making sure that whatever distance you choose, your bent knee does not go past the ankle.

Benefits: Hip mobility, leg strength/flexibility, arm and shoulder strength/mobility, side stretch, core activation, improves balance, builds bone mass, lymphatic drainage in arms, stimulates lymph system, increases heart rate for cardiovascular health

TRIANGLE

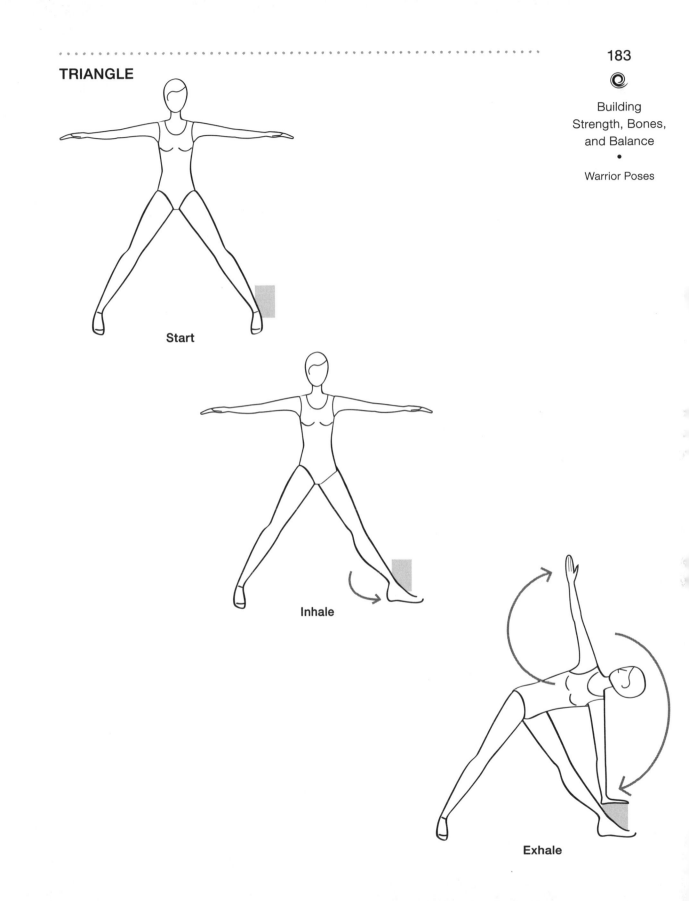

Start

Inhale

Exhale

Balancing Acts

STAND TALL ON ONE FOOT

Props needed: One block or stair step

Stand tall to the right of a block on the lowest level (or a stair step).

INHALE: Place your left foot on the block. Keep your gaze looking straight ahead.

EXHALE: Shift weight into the left foot, straightening the leg. Leave your right toes in contact with the floor if needed for balance. If you are stable enough, experiment with swinging your right foot back and forth while balancing on the left leg.

Hold for ten breaths for optimal bone building.

Repeat on the second side, balancing on the right foot.

Modifications: If balance is challenging for you, you may wish to practice this pose with one hand resting on a wall. Use the opposite hand from the leg that is being lifted.

Benefits: Builds bone mass; strengthens legs, feet and core; improves balance, releases tension in hips

STAND TALL ON ONE FOOT

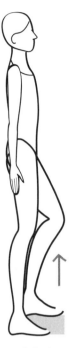

Inhale

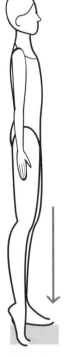

Exhale

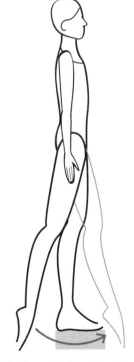

**Optional intensification,
swing foot back and forth**

WARRIOR THREE AT THE WALL

Props needed: Wall, table, or stable chair with a high back

Begin in Down Dog at the Wall (page 166), or rest your hands on a chair back or table instead of the wall.

INHALE: Slightly bend your right knee. Lift and straighten your left leg back behind you, maintaining a neutral spine.

EXHALE: Press your right foot into the floor and straighten your right leg. Engage your abdominal muscles to support your spine. Reach the crown of your head toward the wall while reaching back with your left heel, toes flexed downward. Notice if one hip is lifting higher than the other and try to make the hips even.

Optionally:

INHALE: Reach your right arm straight back alongside your right hip, palm facing the hip.

EXHALE: Reach your left arm back alongside your left hip so that you are now balancing in Warrior Three.

Hold for three breaths. As you inhale, lengthen from the crown of your head to your lifted heel. As you exhale, root down through your standing foot. To release from the pose, bring your hands back to the wall. Lower your left foot to the floor and walk toward the wall to come up to stand.

Repeat on the second side, reaching the right leg back.

Modifications: Tightness in your legs or hips may not allow you to fully straighten your legs in this pose. Modify with knees slightly bent throughout the sequence. If you feel too much stress in your shoulders or chest, try bringing your hands a little above hip height on the wall. Make sure you are not dropping your head toward the floor, which puts more stress on the shoulders. The lifted leg does not have to be at hip height. Lift it as high as you are able (never above hip height) while keeping it straight.

Benefits: Builds bone mass; strengthens the whole body including core, legs, hips, shoulders, arms, and back muscles; increases leg flexibility; stimulates the lymph system; increases heart rate for cardiovascular health

WARRIOR THREE AT THE WALL

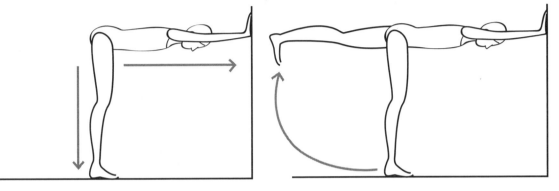

Inhale

Exhale

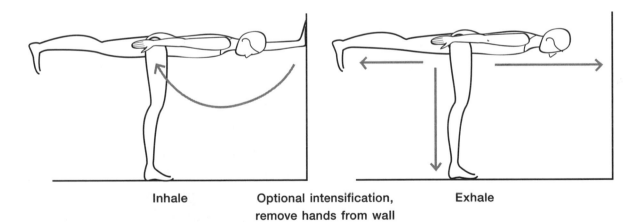

Inhale

Optional intensification,
remove hands from wall

Exhale

FREE WARRIOR THREE

Props needed: Two blocks or stable chair

Place two blocks on the highest level, shoulder width apart. It may be helpful to stack two blocks on top of each other as shown in the illustration, or use a chair instead.

Stand tall approximately eighteen inches behind the blocks.

INHALE: Sweep your arms out and up like swan wings.

EXHALE: Bend forward from your hips and bring your hands onto the blocks. Keep your spine long, reaching the crown of your head forward. Avoid rounding your spine or dropping your head. If your head is below your hips, add more support under your hands.

INHALE: Lift your straight left leg up and back, keeping your hips level. Flex your left toes downward.

Optionally:

INHALE: Reach your straight right arm forward alongside your ear, palm facing in toward your head.

Hold for three breaths. As you inhale bend your right leg slightly. Lengthen from the crown of your head (and your extended arm) to your lifted heel. As you exhale straighten your right leg. Engage your core by drawing your navel toward your spine.

Repeat on the second side.

Modifications: Tightness in your legs or hips may not allow you to fully straighten your legs in this pose. Modify with knees slightly bent throughout the sequence. If you feel too much stress in your shoulders or chest, try bringing your hands a little above hip height on the wall. Make sure you are not dropping your head toward the floor, which puts more stress on the shoulders. The lifted leg does not have to be at hip height. Lift it as high as you are able (never above hip height) while keeping it straight.

Benefits: Builds bone mass; strengthens the whole body including core, legs, hips, shoulders, arms, and back muscles; increases leg flexibility; stimulates the lymph system; increases heart rate for cardiovascular health

FREE WARRIOR THREE

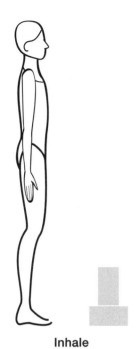

Inhale

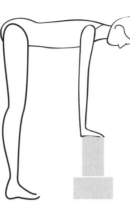

Exhale

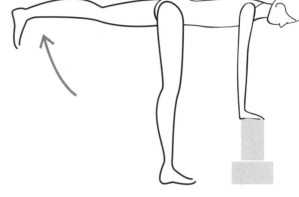

Inhale

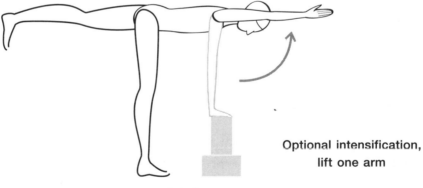

Inhale

**Optional intensification,
lift one arm**

REST AND RESTORE

Restorative Poses

The physical challenge of restorative poses is to find a position that allows your body to release tension and fully relax. Props should be used to ensure every part of your body is comfortable and supported. Adjust all props as needed for your body. Warmth, darkness, and quiet promote rest, so you may want to cover up with a blanket and turn off the lights, also making sure to turn off your phone. Once you have set yourself up in a restorative pose, commit to stillness.

RESTORATIVE SHOULDERSTAND

Props needed: Two blocks, two blankets, bolster, eye pillow (optional), strap (optional)

Place your bolster in the middle of your mat so the long side of the bolster is parallel with the long side of your mat. Put two blocks at the bottom (foot end) of your mat, and two folded blankets, one on either side of the top part (head end) of your mat (see "How can I support my arms in a cactus shape?" on page 143).

Sit in the middle of the bolster, facing the blocks. Place the blocks on the highest level, one leg length away from the bolster. Make sure the blocks are higher than the bolster (if you have a very large bolster or small blocks, you may need additional props—see Modifications).

Using your arms for support, lower your upper body to the floor so your head and shoulders rest on the mat. Straighten your legs one at a time, resting your ankles/calves on the blocks, heels hanging off. Bring your arms into a cactus shape with forearms resting on the folded blankets.

Close your eyes. Rest for at least five minutes.

Modifications: Limited mobility in your shoulders or chest may require additional blankets under your Cactus arms. Ensure that your hands, wrist, forearms, and elbows are all supported. As always, support both arms at the same height to maintain body symmetry. For neck support, place a small blanket roll under your neck. If your neck feels strained, a low pillow under the head can offer additional support. A yoga strap can be belted around your thighs to hold your legs in place and allow the legs to fully relax. If you have two bolsters or additional blankets, place them on top of the blocks to create a softer support for your ankles/calves. In this case the blocks may need to be on a lower level, but make sure your ankles remain higher than your hips.

RESTORATIVE SHOULDERSTAND

Benefits: Lymphatic drainage from legs, pelvis, and abdomen; increases venous return from the lower body; chest opening; activates the parasympathetic nervous system, promoting physical relaxation, calm, and stress reduction

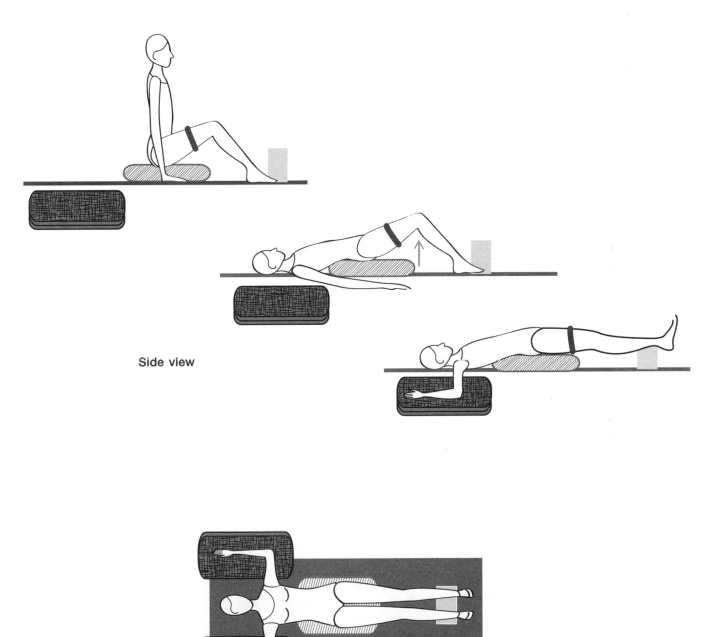

Side view

Top view

RESTORATIVE COBBLER

Props needed: Bolster, blanket (or cushion), two blocks, eye pillow (optional), additional blankets (optional)

Place your bolster in the middle of your mat so the long side of the bolster is parallel with the long side of your mat. Put a folded blanket (or cushion) on the end of the bolster that is closer to the top (head end) of the mat. Make sure your blocks are within reach.

Sit in front of the bolster at the bottom of the mat so that your hips are up against the end, the shorter side, of the bolster (do not sit on the bolster). Bend your knees, placing the soles of your feet together, dropping your knees apart so your legs make a diamond shape. Place a block under each knee or thigh at a height that fully supports the weight of each leg.

Lower your upper body onto the bolster, head and neck supported by the folded blanket. Extend your arms out to either side of the bolster, palms facing up.

Close your eyes. Rest for at least five minutes.

Modifications: If your chest feels overstretched or your arms are uncomfortable, use additional folded blankets under your arms, supporting forearms and hands.

Benefits: Chest opening; activates the parasympathetic nervous system, promoting physical relaxation, calm, and stress reduction

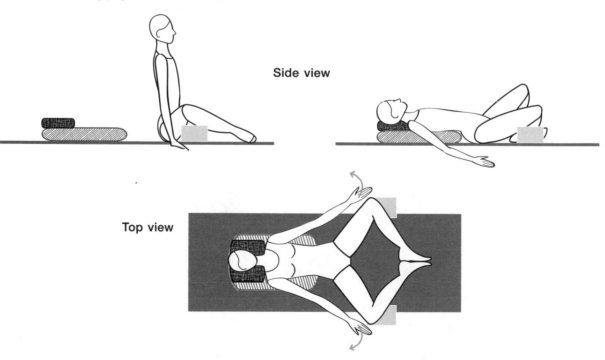

Side view

Top view

Tips for Restorative Poses

Why is symmetry important?

While our bodies are never perfectly symmetrical, moving the body in a symmetrical way, or using props to support the body in a symmetrical position, promotes muscle relaxation and balance. If one of your shoulders is more mobile than the other, you may notice in a pose like Swan Wings that one arm is able to lift higher than the other, or in Restorative Fish that one arm easily rests on the blanket while the other hovers above. Similarly, if one hip is more flexible than the other, in Restorative Cobbler one knee may easily rest on a low block, while the other does not. However challenging it may be to accept what we see as our limitations, it is important to align the yoga poses in a symmetrical way, guided by the body's less mobile, less flexible side. In Swan Wings, lift both arms to the same height, even if one arm is able to go higher. In Restorative Cobbler, support both knees at the height required for the comfort of the less flexible side of your body.

How can I best support my neck?

The position of your head and neck in rest and restore poses may determine whether the rest of your body is able to fully relax. Once you have set yourself up in the pose, notice whether your chin is jutting up toward the ceiling and/or the back of your neck feels shortened or compressed. If so, use additional props such as a folded blanket or small pillow to support your head and neck so that your forehead is slightly higher than your chin. This can sometimes also be achieved without any additional props, simply by adjusting the alignment of your head so the back of your neck elongates and your chin drops. Once your neck is released and relaxed, the rest of your body is more likely to follow.

Why use an eye pillow?

Darkness promotes rest. In all rest and restore poses, using an eye pillow to cover your eyes can be beneficial, offering soothing darkness, helping the eye muscles to fully relax, and putting gentle pressure on the eyes and forehead that can help to quiet the mind.

LEGS UP THE WALL

Props needed: Wall, two blankets, eye pillow (optional), bolster/cushion (optional), strap (optional), additional blanket (optional)

Pull the short end of your yoga mat up to a wall. Place a folded blanket on either side of the middle of your mat.

Sit facing the long side of the mat with your left shoulder against the wall, knees bent.

Using your right arm for support, lie down on your right side and as you roll onto your back, extend both legs up the wall. Keep your hips several inches away from the wall. Rest your arms on the folded blankets in a cactus shape (see "How can I support my arms in a cactus shape?" on page 143).

Close your eyes. Rest for at least five minutes.

Modifications: If your neck feels strained, a folded blanket or low pillow under the head can offer additional support. If your hamstrings are tight, having your legs up the wall may feel like a stretch, and the back of your hips may not be flat to the floor. Move your hips further away from the wall until they rest fully on the mat. This will also release tension in the backs of the legs. Limited mobility in your shoulders or chest may require additional blankets under your Cactus arms. Ensure that your hands, wrist, forearms, and elbows are all supported. As always, support both arms at the same height to maintain body symmetry. Optionally, put a bolster (with long end parallel to the wall) or cushion under your hips. A yoga strap can be belted around your thighs to hold your legs in place and allow the legs to more fully relax.

Benefits: Lymphatic drainage from legs; increases venous return from the lower body; activates the parasympathetic nervous system, promoting physical relaxation, calm, and stress reduction

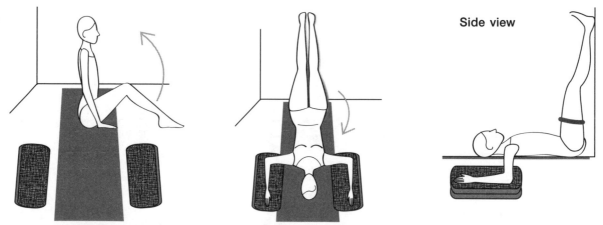

Top view   **Side view**

RESTORATIVE FISH

Props needed: Two blankets, two blocks, eye pillow (optional)

At the back of and parallel to the short side of your mat, place one block on the middle level. Place a second block on the lowest level approximately twelve inches in front of the first. Set the folded blankets on either side of the top end of the mat (see "How can I support my arms in a cactus shape?" on page 143).

Sit in the middle of the mat, facing away from the blocks. Bend your knees, placing the soles of your feet on the floor. Use your arms for support to lower your upper body onto the blocks.

Rest the bottom tips of your shoulder blades on the lower block. Make sure you are not resting your waist or the back of your neck or upper shoulders on this block. Support your head with the higher block. Adjust the location of the blocks as needed.

Extend your legs. Rest your arms on the folded blankets in a cactus shape.

Close your eyes. Rest for at least five minutes.

Modifications: If you feel discomfort in your lower back, bend your knees and place a bolster or rolled-up blanket under them for support. If your head is uncomfortable resting on the block, put a blanket or towel over the block for extra cushioning. Limited mobility in your shoulders or chest may require additional blankets under your Cactus arms. Ensure that your hands, wrist, forearms, and elbows are all supported. As always, support both arms at the same height to maintain body symmetry.

Benefits: Chest opening; increases range of motion in shoulders and arms; improves upper spine flexibility; activates the parasympathetic nervous system, promoting physical relaxation, calm, and stress reduction

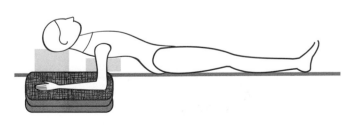

Side view

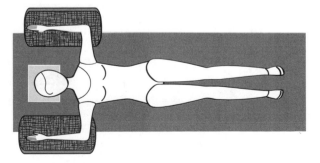

Top view

RESTORATIVE BRIDGE

Props needed: One block, two blankets, eye pillow (optional)

Set the folded blankets on either side of the top end of the mat (see "How can I support my arms in a cactus shape?" on page 143). Have the block within reach.

Lie down on your back. Bend your knees, bringing your feet to the floor, hip width apart. Rest your arms alongside your body, palms down.

Press your feet and arms into the floor in order to lift your hips up. Slide a block under your hips on the lowest level in a horizontal position so that both hips can be supported. Rest your arms on the folded blankets in a cactus shape.

Close your eyes. Rest for at least five minutes.

Modifications: If the block is too high to fit under your hips, use a folded blanket or cushion instead. Make sure your hips (sacrum), not your spine or waist, are resting on the support. If your neck feels strained, a folded blanket or low pillow under the head can offer additional support (see "How can I best support my neck?" on page 193). Limited mobility in your shoulders or chest may require additional blankets under your Cactus arms. Ensure that your hands, wrist, forearms, and elbows are all supported. As always, support both arms at the same height to maintain body symmetry.

Benefits: Chest opening; increases range of motion in shoulders and arms; improves spine flexibility; lymphatic drainage from pelvis and abdomen; activates the parasympathetic nervous system, promoting physical relaxation, calm, and stress reduction

SAVASANA/SUNSET POSE

Optional props: Blankets, eye pillow, bolster

Lie on your back. Extend your legs and separate them slightly. Rest your arms a little bit away from your sides, palms facing up. Make sure your body is not touching any other props or objects that are not supporting the pose.

Feel the back surface of your body resting on the floor. Make any adjustments that would allow your hips, spine, shoulders, head, and neck to rest in a neutral, comfortable position.

Close your eyes. As you exhale, release the weight of your body into the floor. Rest for at least five minutes.

Modifications: Place a folded blanket under your head and neck if your neck feels uncomfortable. Put a bolster or rolled-up blanket under your knees to release lower back tension.

Benefits: Activates the parasympathetic nervous system, promoting physical relaxation, calm, and stress reduction

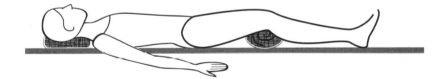

Side view

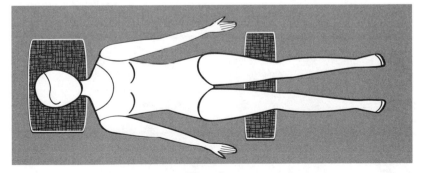

Top view

*It is solely by risking life
that freedom is obtained.*

GEORG WILHELM FRIEDRICH HEGEL

Patricia, cancer survivor

7

Sample Practices for Varying Stages of Your Treatment and Recovery

This chapter offers sample sequences based on various levels and time lengths so that you have the flexibility to choose a sequence depending on how you are feeling on any given day. They are designed to be effective for both new and experienced yoga practitioners. The individual poses introduced in the previous pages are carefully sequenced into a complete practice. If you are a cancer survivor in treatment, in recovery, maintaining your new normal, or gaining new strength, these samplers are a way to structure your home practice. Or if you are a yoga teacher for cancer patients or survivors, you can use these sample sequences as a basic outline to help plan your classes.

Developing an effective and safe home practice: Going to a group yoga class has many benefits, but a home practice can be more practical for a busy schedule and more tailored to your individual needs, empowering you to manage your own wellness plan as well as offering a different set of profound insights. Whether you are brand new to yoga, or have been practicing for many years, a home practice challenges you to listen closely each day to what your body requires.

Fear is a normal response to cancer. How to manage both is the question.

TARI PRINSTER

Your body is your teacher! Be inquisitive about how each pose feels and you will develop intuition about what yoga poses you want and need to do on any given day. For example, an advanced yoga practitioner who is feeling fatigued might be wise to choose a more restorative "In Treatment" sequence. A survivor who is in treatment but feeling strong might wish to jump to a more energizing "In Recovery" or "Maintaining the New Normal" sequence. As you explore what you need with a sense of curiosity and creativity, allow yourself to be spontaneous. These sequences are simply a framework. The attention you bring to them—awareness and curiosity about your physical sensations, breath, emotions, and thoughts—is the practice.

IN TREATMENT—30 MINUTES

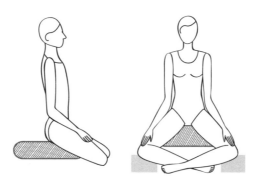

Dynamic Stillness/Breathing/Meditation (pages 115–22)

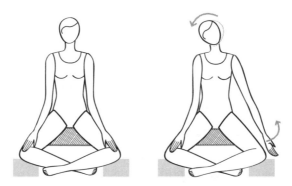

Neck Stretch (page 124)

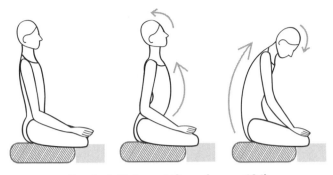

Seated Cat and Cow (page 131)

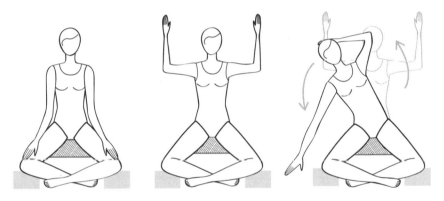

Cactus Teapot (page 129)

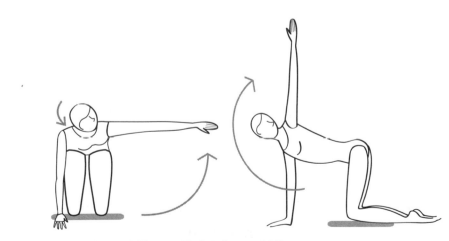

Hands and Knees Twist (page 146)
(see arm modification on page 147 if needed)

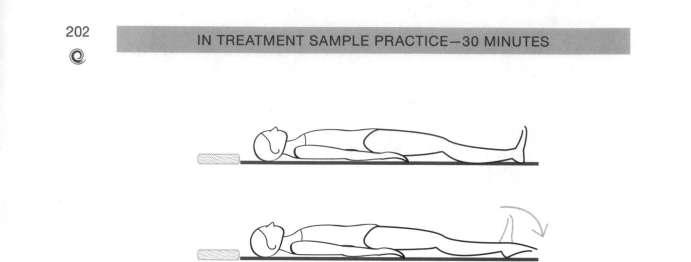

Part 1, just feet

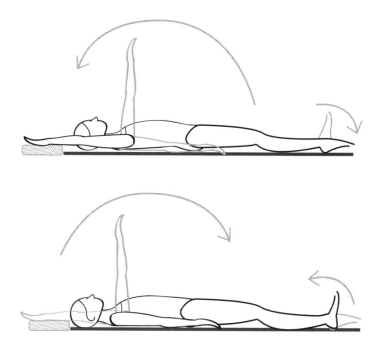

Part 2, with arms

Full-Body Stretch (page 134)

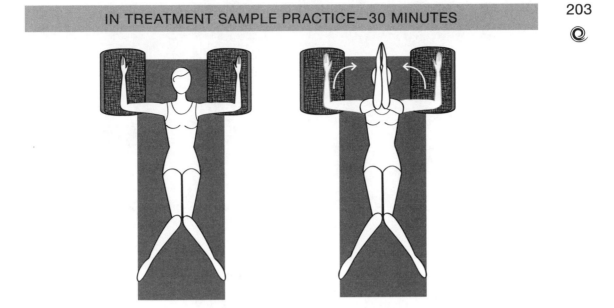

Knock-Kneed Cactus Clap (page 141)

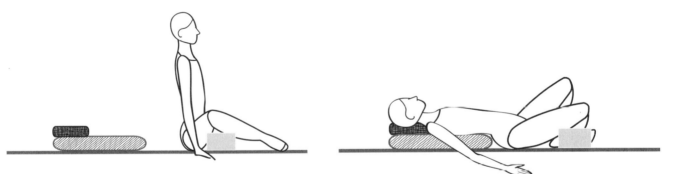

Restorative Cobbler (page 192)

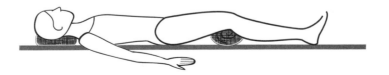

Savasana/Sunset Pose (page 197)

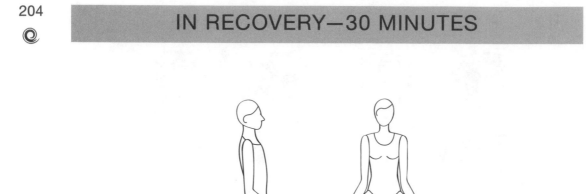

Dynamic Stillness/Breathing/Meditation (pages 115–22)

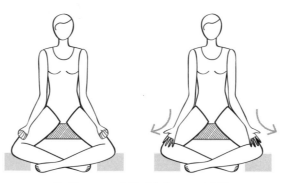

Gather and Hold (page 125)

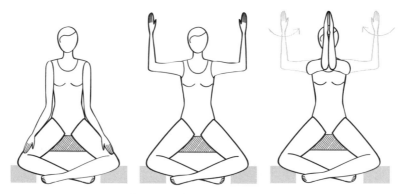

Cactus Clap (page 127)

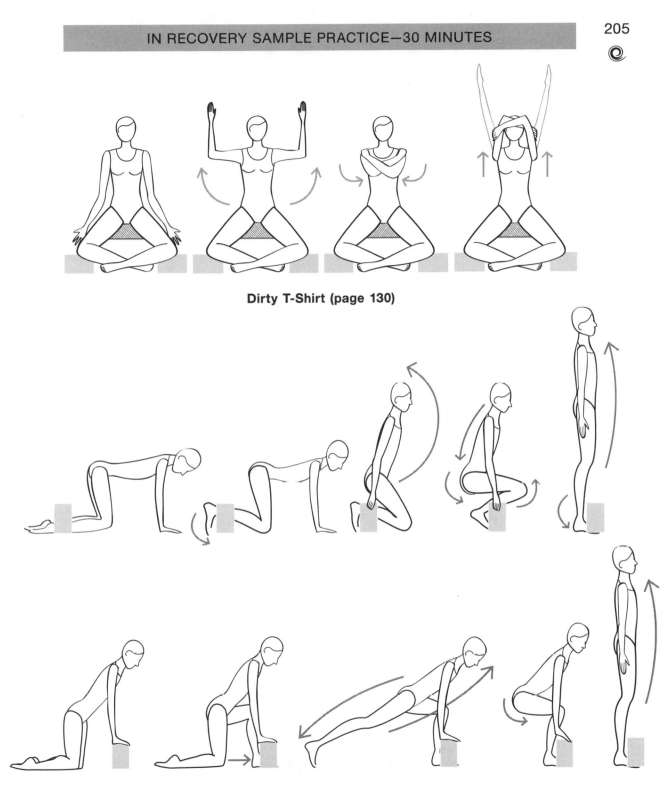

Dirty T-Shirt (page 130)

Toe Massage to Stand (top) or Lunge to Stand (bottom)
(pages 158 and 160)

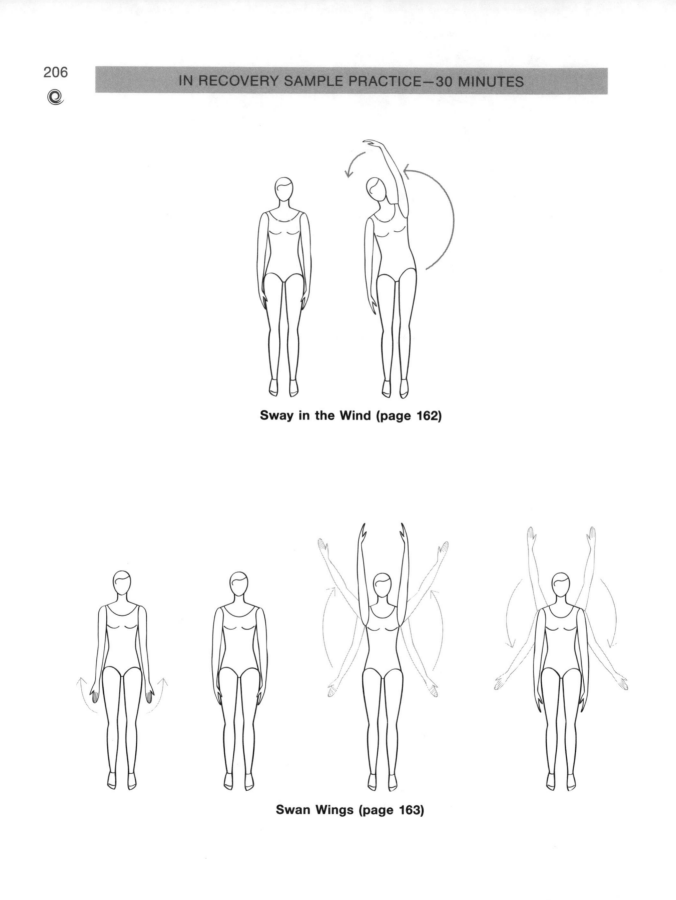

Sway in the Wind (page 162)

Swan Wings (page 163)

IN RECOVERY SAMPLE PRACTICE—30 MINUTES

Part 1, legs only

Part 2, with head turns

Leg Rocking (page 136)

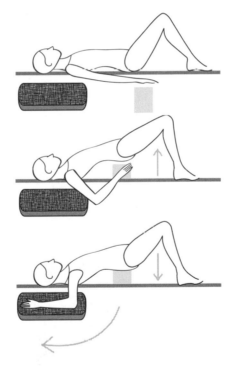

Restorative Bridge (page 196)

Savasana/Sunset Pose (page 197)

MAINTAINING THE NEW NORMAL—
30 MINUTES

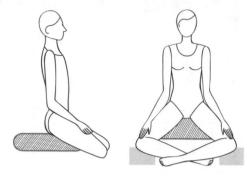

Dynamic Stillness/Breathing/Meditation (pages 115–22)

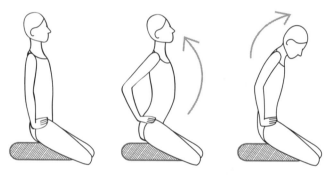

Pelvic Tilt (page 123)

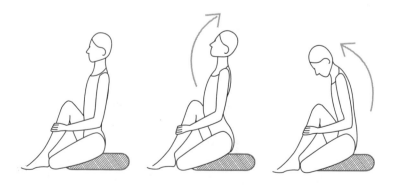

Knee-Up Seated Cat and Cow (page 132)

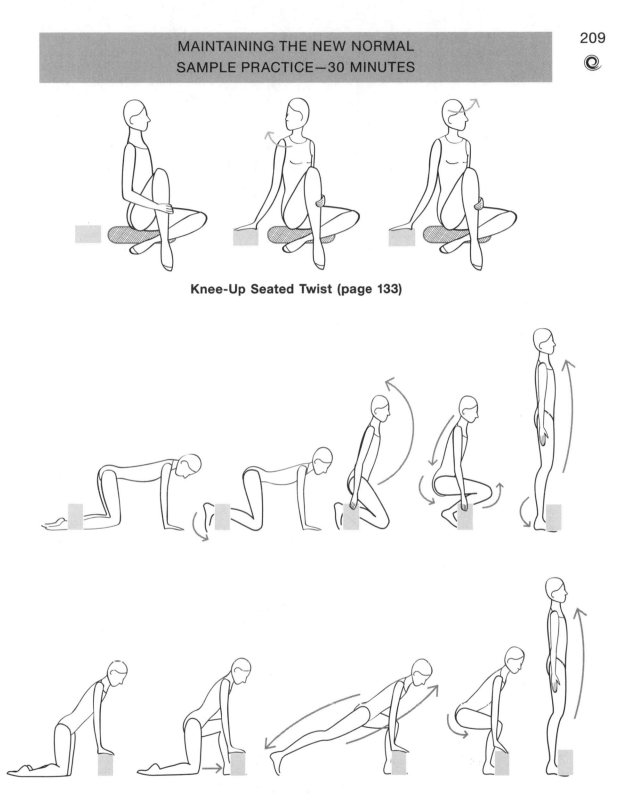

Knee-Up Seated Twist (page 133)

**Toe Massage to Stand (top) or Lunge to Stand (bottom)
(pages 158 and 160)**

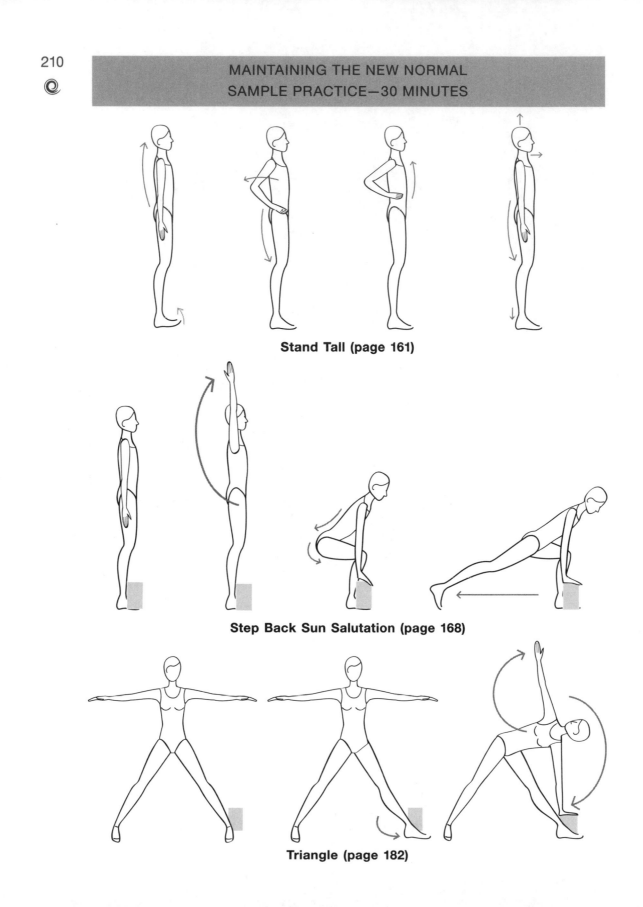

Stand Tall (page 161)

Step Back Sun Salutation (page 168)

Triangle (page 182)

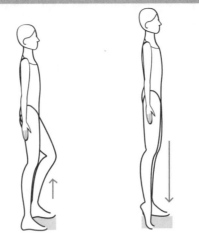

Stand Tall on One Foot (page 184)
(see optional intensification on page 185 if needed)

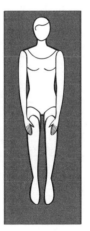 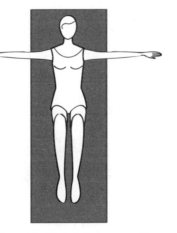

Crunch Twist (page 140)

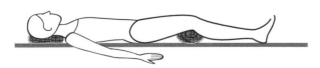

Savasana/Sunset Pose (page 197)

GAINING STRENGTH
SAMPLE PRACTICE—30 MINUTES

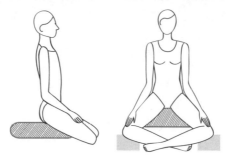

Dynamic Stillness/Breathing/Meditation (pages 115–22)

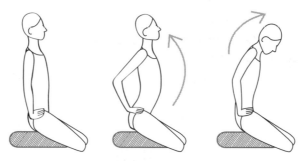

Pelvic Tilt (page 123)

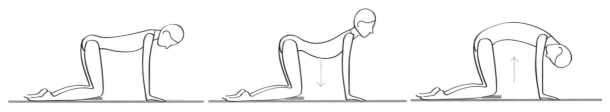

Cat and Cow (page 145)

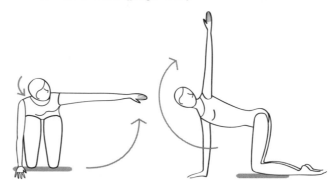

Hands and Knees Twist (page 146)
(see arm modification on page 147 if needed)

GAINING STRENGTH
SAMPLE PRACTICE—30 MINUTES

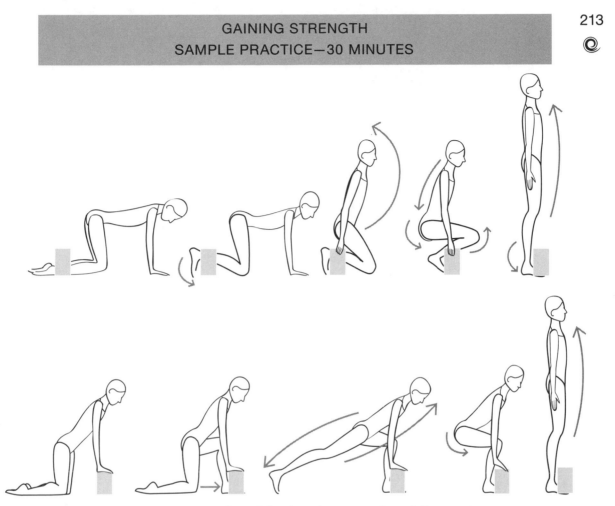

**Toe Massage to Stand (top) or Lunge to Stand (bottom)
(pages 158 and 160)**

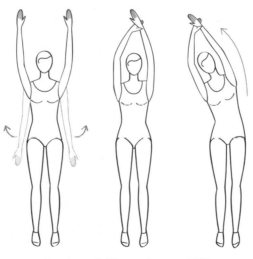

Crescent Moon (page 165)

GAINING STRENGTH
SAMPLE PRACTICE—30 MINUTES

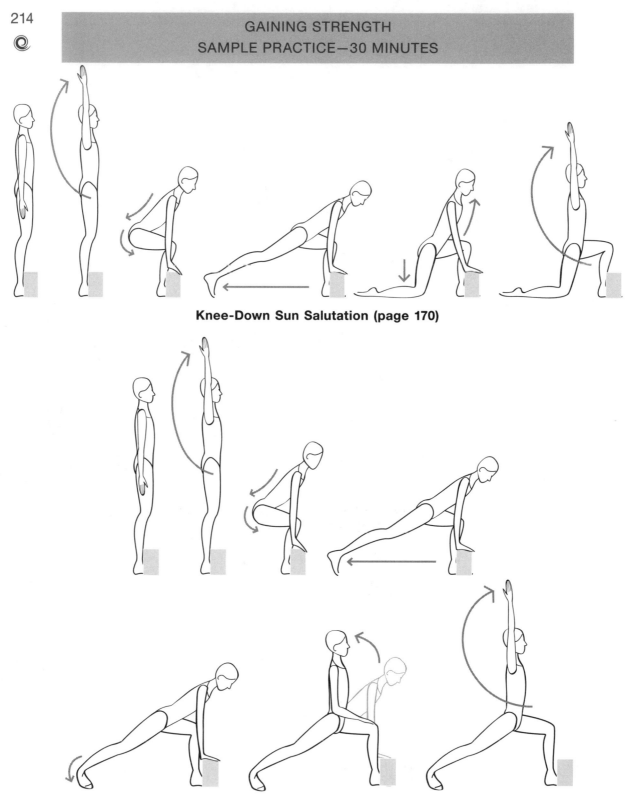

Knee-Down Sun Salutation (page 170)

Warrior One (page 176)

GAINING STRENGTH
SAMPLE PRACTICE—30 MINUTES

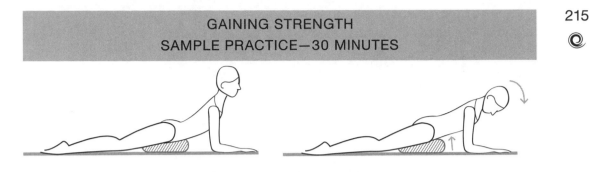

Slumber Party (page 155)

Part 1, legs only   Part 2, with head lifts

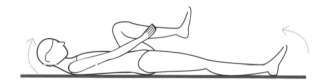

Crunch and Switch (page 138)

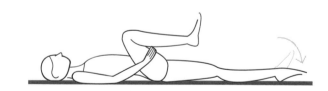

Savasana/Sunset Pose (page 197)

IN TREATMENT—60 MINUTES

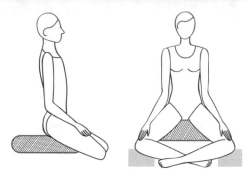

Dynamic Stillness/Breathing/Meditation (pages 115–22)

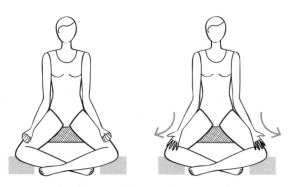

Gather and Hold (page 125)

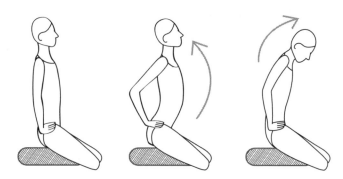

Pelvic Tilt (page 123)

Cat and Cow (page 145)

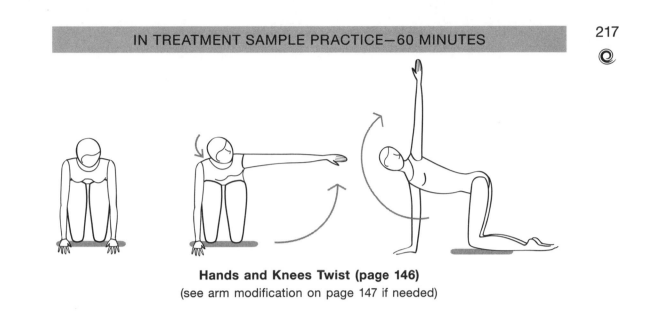

Hands and Knees Twist (page 146)

(see arm modification on page 147 if needed)

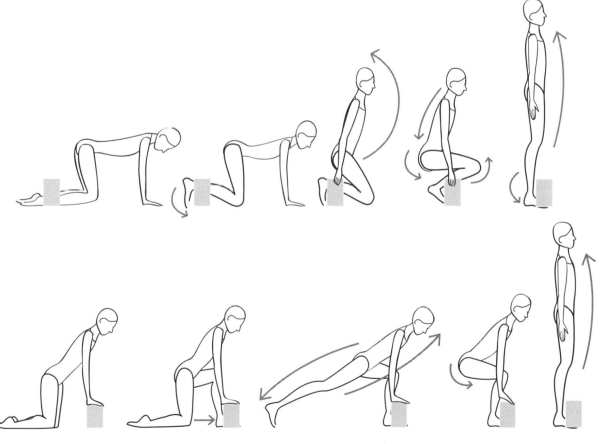

Toe Massage to Stand (top) or Lunge to Stand (bottom)
(pages 158 and 160)

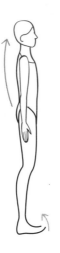
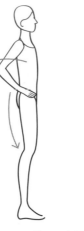
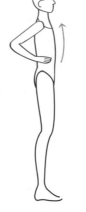
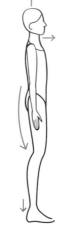

Stand Tall (page 161)

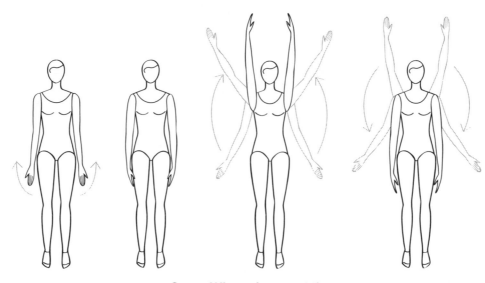

Swan Wings (page 163)

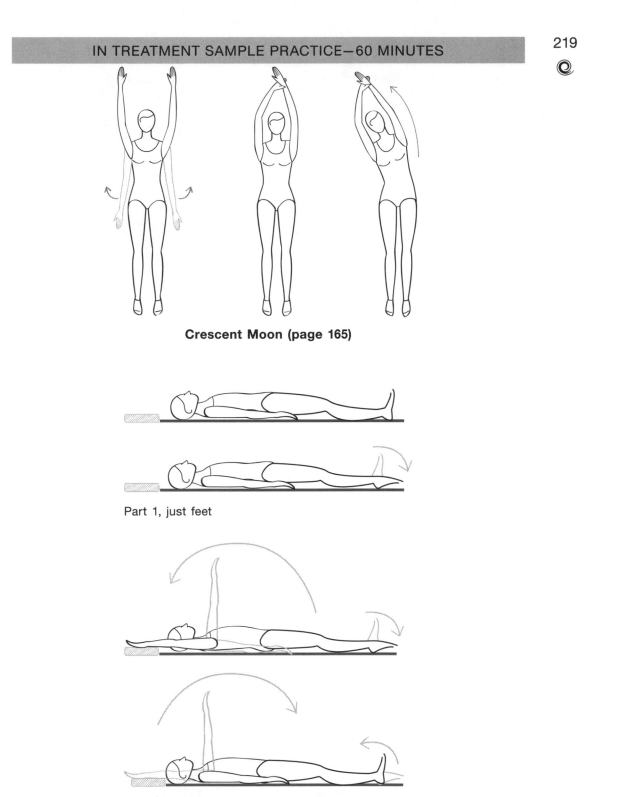

Crescent Moon (page 165)

Part 1, just feet

Part 2, with arms

Full-Body Stretch (page 134)

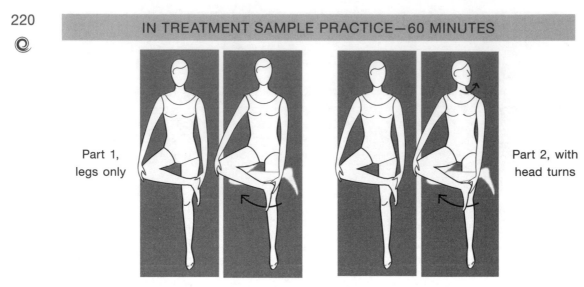

Part 1, legs only

Part 2, with head turns

Leg Rocking (page 136)

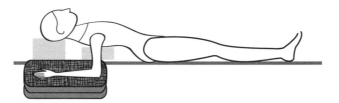

Restorative Fish (page 195)

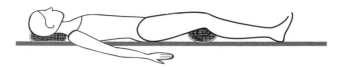

Savasana/Sunset Pose (page 197)

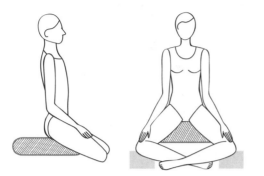

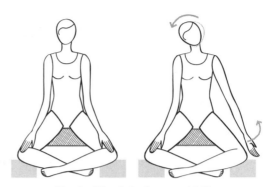

**Dynamic Stillness/Breathing/Meditation
(pages 115–22)**

Neck Stretch (page 124)

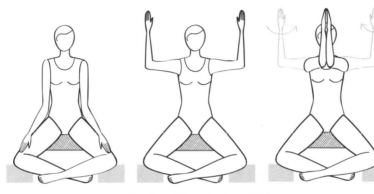

Cactus Clap (page 127)

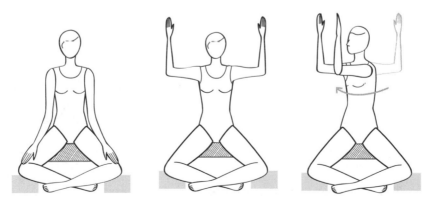

Cactus Twist (page 128)

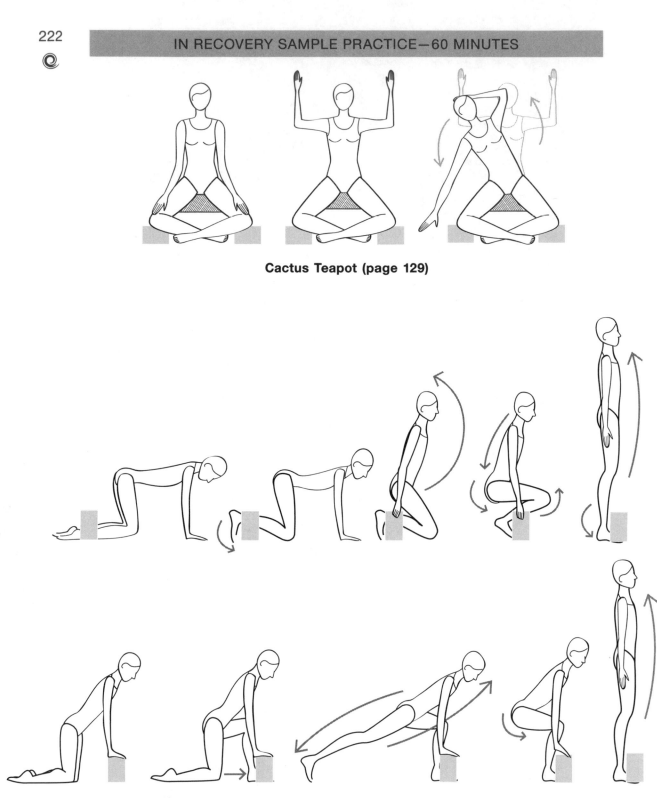

Cactus Teapot (page 129)

**Toe Massage to Stand (top) or Lunge to Stand (bottom)
(pages 158 and 160)**

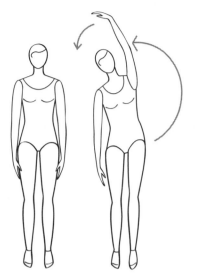

**Sway in the Wind
(page 162)**

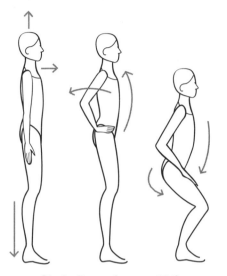

Chair Pose (page 164)

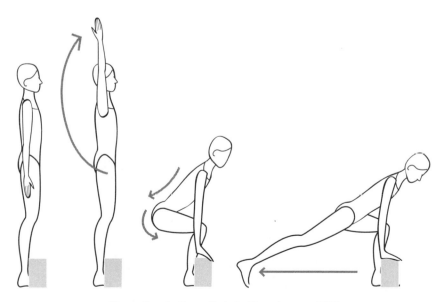

Step Back Sun Salutation (page 168)

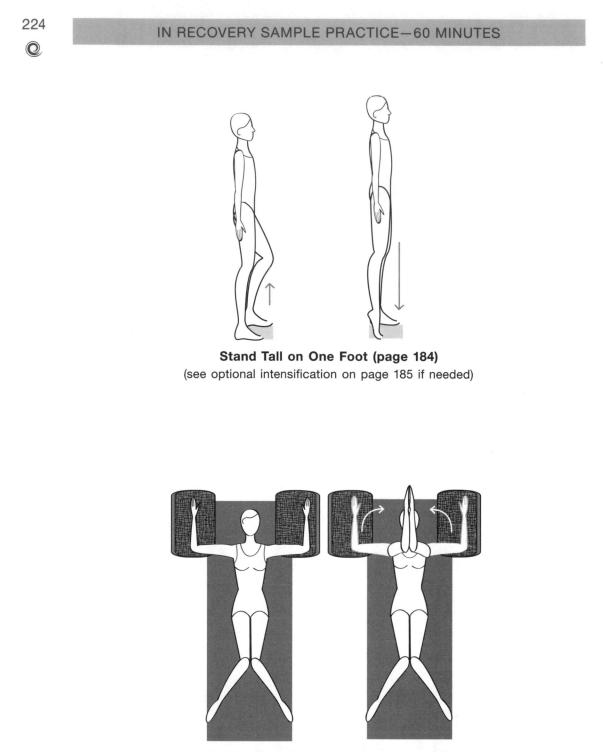

Stand Tall on One Foot (page 184)
(see optional intensification on page 185 if needed)

Knock-Kneed Cactus Clap (page 141)

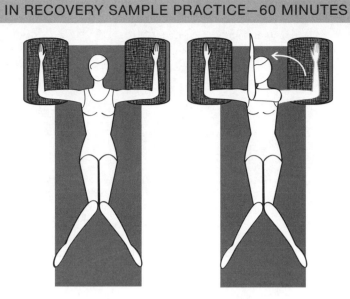

Knock-Kneed Cactus Twist (page 142)

Restorative Cobbler (page 192)

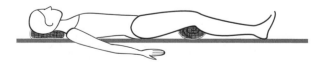

Savasana/Sunset Pose (page 197)

MAINTAINING THE NEW NORMAL—
60 MINUTES

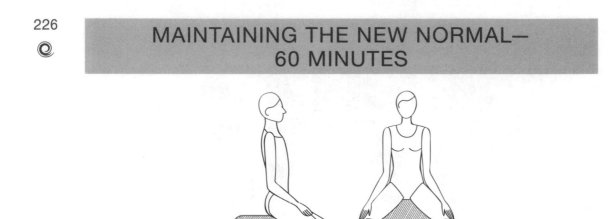

Dynamic Stillness/Breathing/Meditation (pages 115–22)

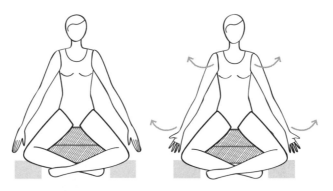

Thumbs-Up (page 126)

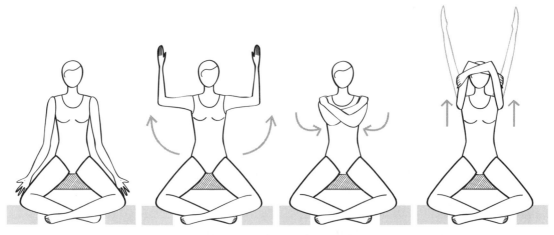

Dirty T-Shirt (page 130)

Twist Extension (page 150)
(see arm modification on page 152 if needed)

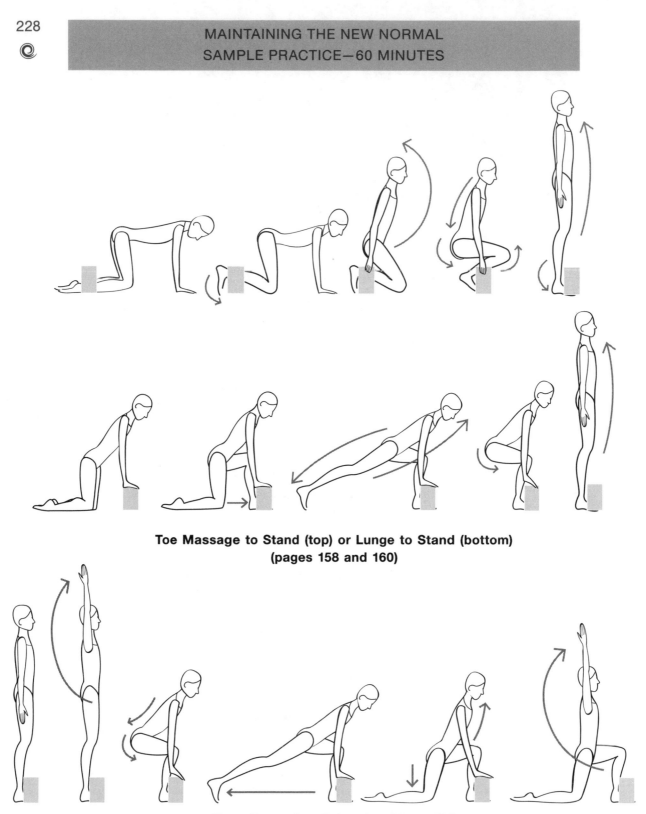

**Toe Massage to Stand (top) or Lunge to Stand (bottom)
(pages 158 and 160)**

Knee-Down Sun Salutation (page 170)

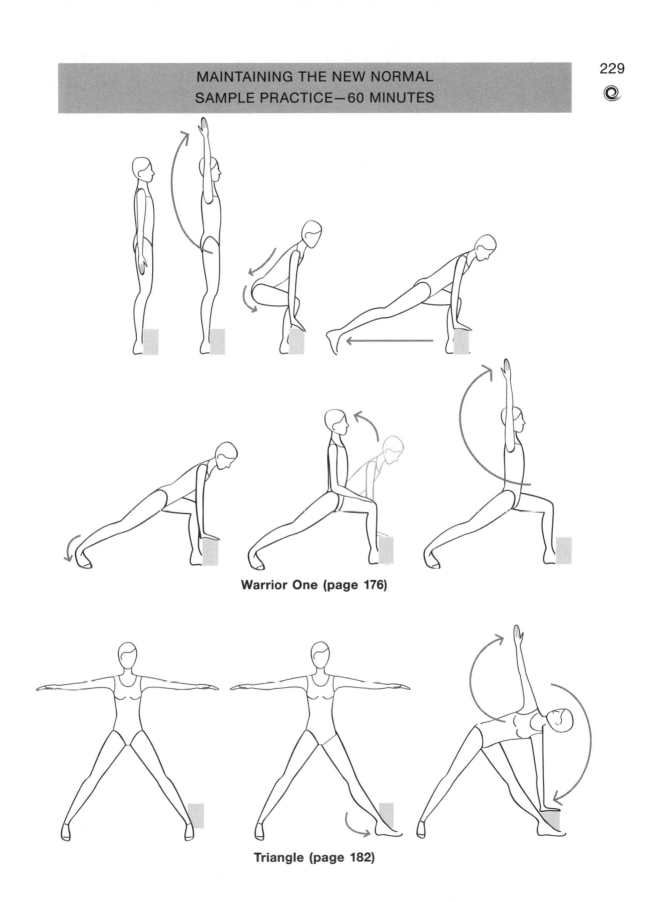

Warrior One (page 176)

Triangle (page 182)

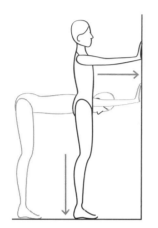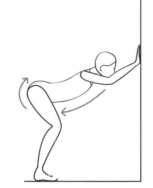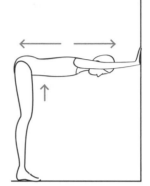

Down Dog at the Wall (page 166)

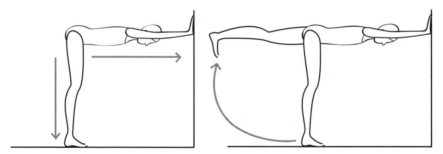

Warrior Three at the Wall (page 186)
(see optional intensification on page 187 if needed)

Slumber Party (page 155)

Part 1, legs only

Part 2, with head lifts

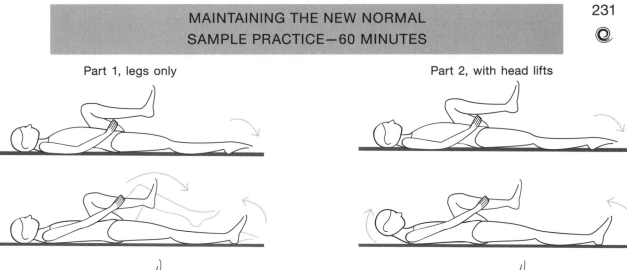

Crunch and Switch (page 138)

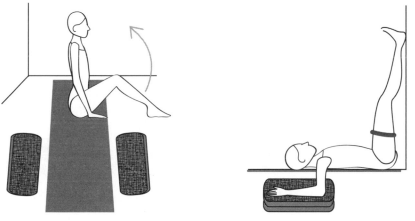

Legs Up the Wall (page 194)

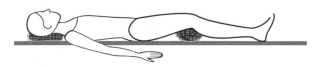

Savasana/Sunset Pose (page 197)

GAINING STRENGTH—60 MINUTES

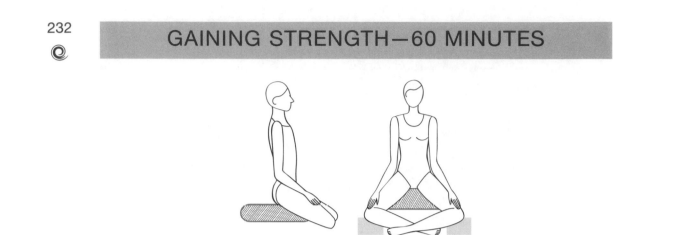

Dynamic Stillness/Breathing/Meditation (pages 115–22)

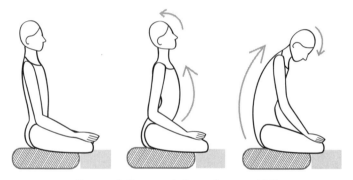

Seated Cat and Cow (page 131)

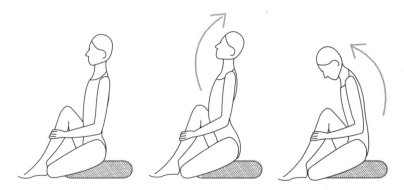

Knee-Up Seated Cat and Cow (page 132)

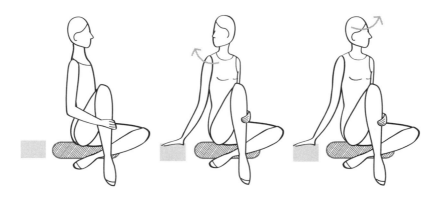

Knee-Up Seated Twist (page 133)

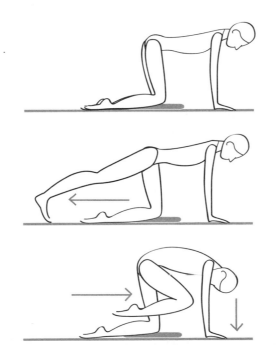

Hands and Knees Leg Extension (page 148)

GAINING STRENGTH
SAMPLE PRACTICE—60 MINUTES

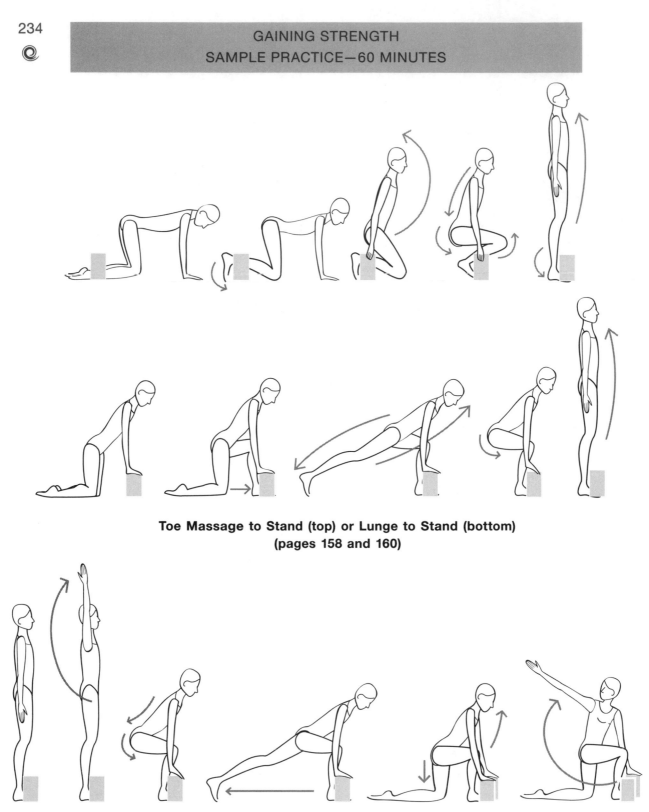

Toe Massage to Stand (top) or Lunge to Stand (bottom)
(pages 158 and 160)

Step Back Twist (page 172)

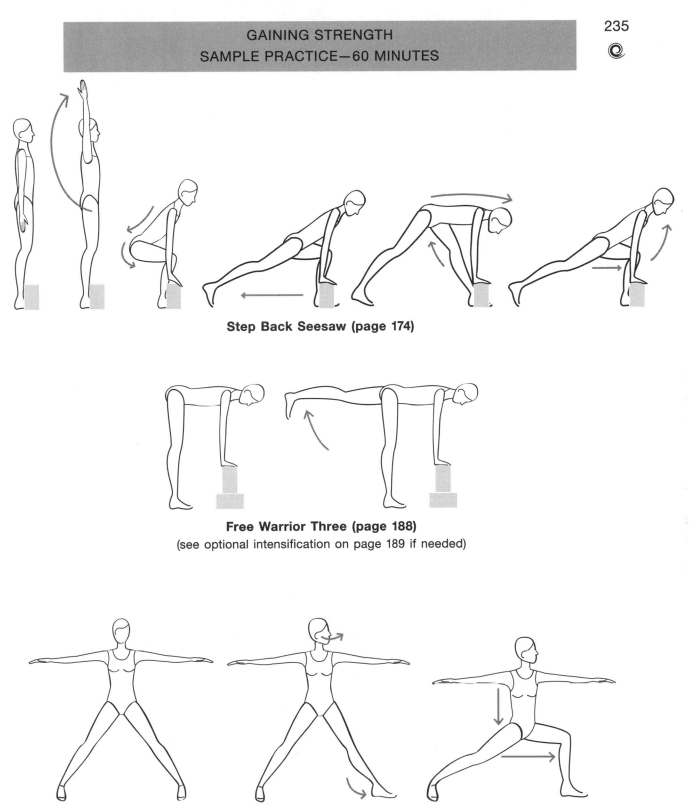

Step Back Seesaw (page 174)

Free Warrior Three (page 188)
(see optional intensification on page 189 if needed)

Warrior Two (page 178)

GAINING STRENGTH
SAMPLE PRACTICE—60 MINUTES

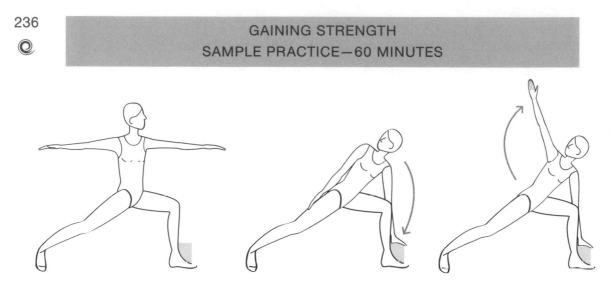

Side Angle (page 180)

(see arm modification on page 181 if needed)

Part 1, warm up kicks   Part 2, with head turn and foot grab

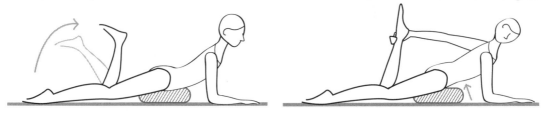

Butt Kick (page 156)

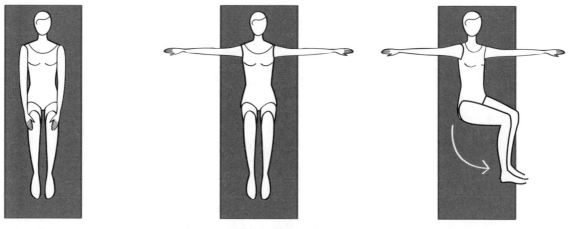

Crunch Twist (page 140)

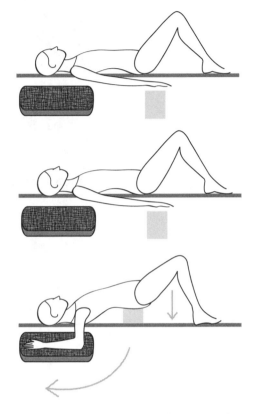

Restorative Bridge (page 196)

Savasana/Sunset Pose (page 197)

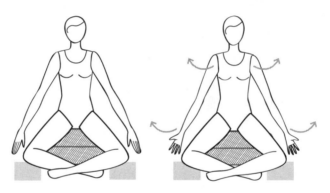

Dynamic Stillness/Breathing/Meditation (pages 115–22)

Thumbs-Up (page 126)

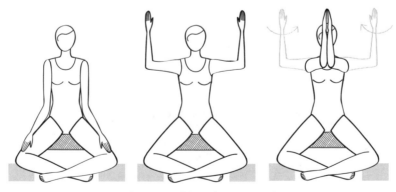

Cactus Clap (page 127)

GAINING STRENGTH
SAMPLE PRACTICE—90 MINUTES

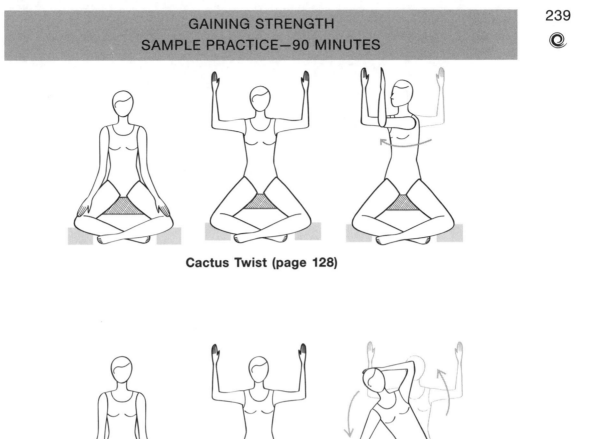

Cactus Twist (page 128)

Cactus Teapot (page 129)

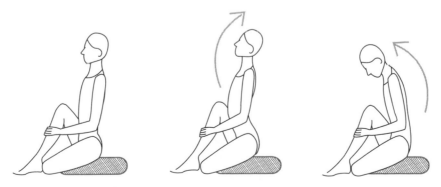

Knee-Up Seated Cat and Cow (page 132)

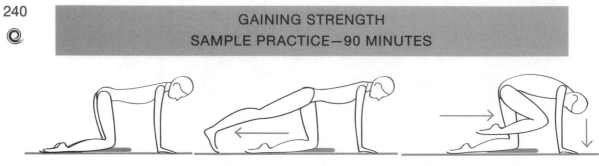

Hands and Knees Leg Extension (page 148)

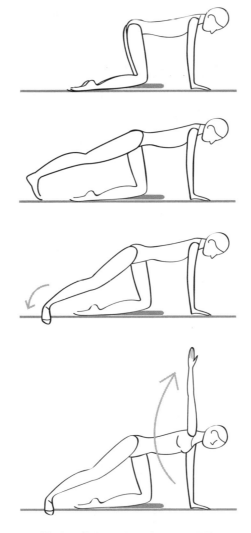

Twist Extension (page 150)
(see arm modification on page 152 if needed)

GAINING STRENGTH
SAMPLE PRACTICE—90 MINUTES

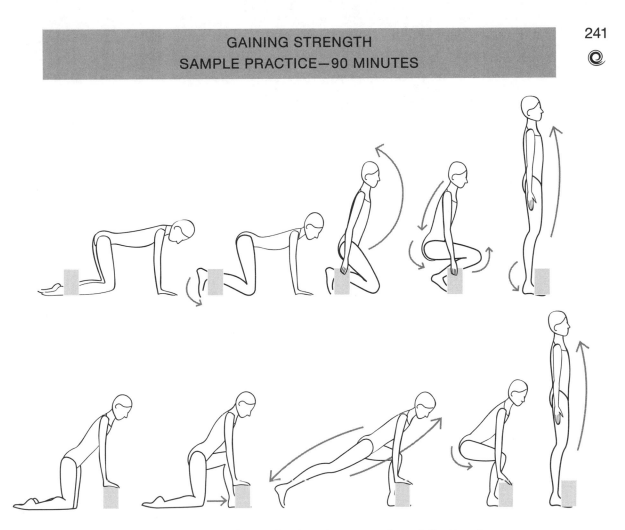

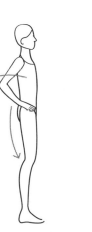

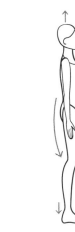

**Toe Massage to Stand (top) or Lunge to Stand (bottom)
(pages 158 and 160)**

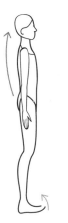

Stand Tall (page 161)

GAINING STRENGTH
SAMPLE PRACTICE—90 MINUTES

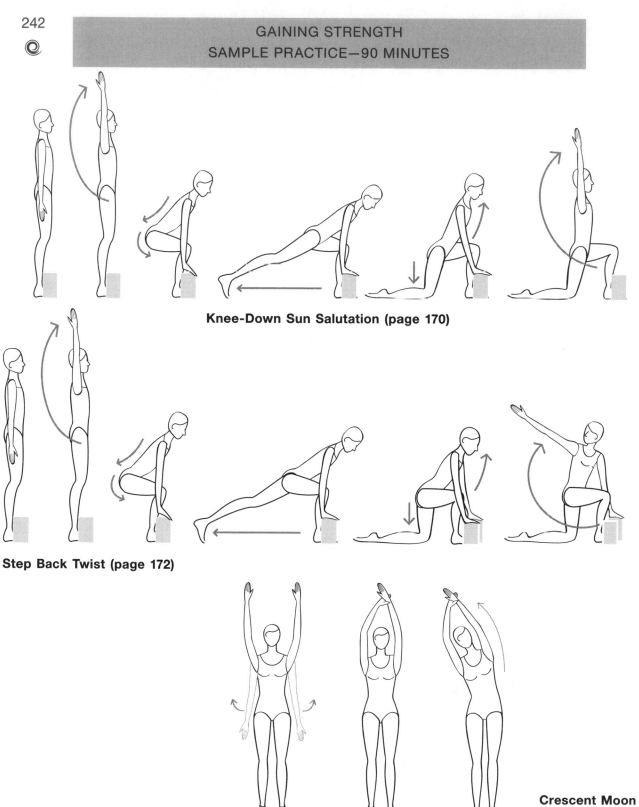

Knee-Down Sun Salutation (page 170)

Step Back Twist (page 172)

**Crescent Moon
(page 165)**

GAINING STRENGTH
SAMPLE PRACTICE—90 MINUTES

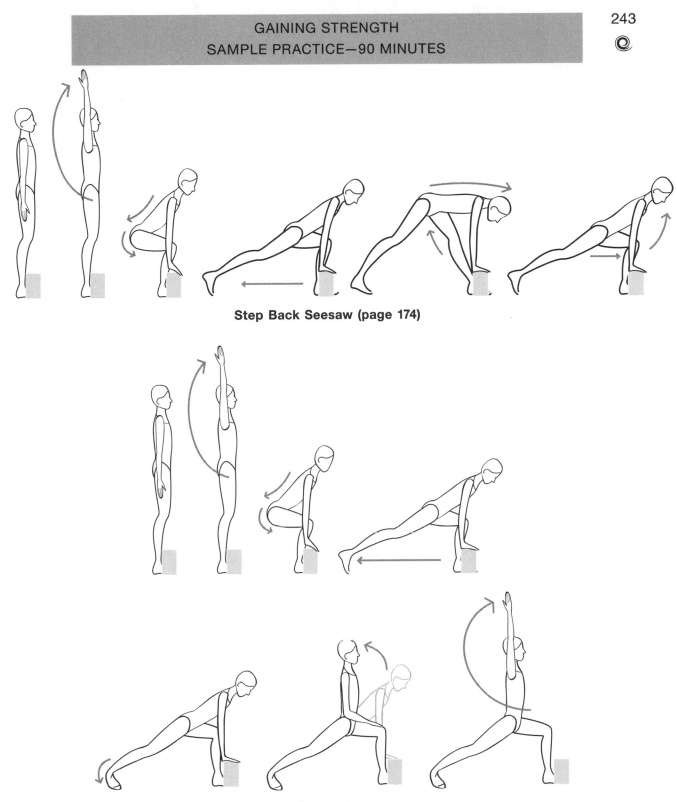

Step Back Seesaw (page 174)

Warrior One (page 176)

GAINING STRENGTH
SAMPLE PRACTICE—90 MINUTES

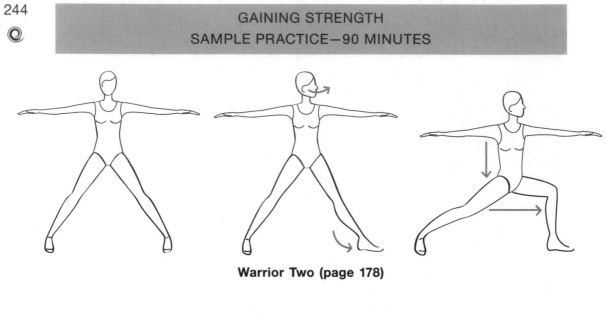

Warrior Two (page 178)

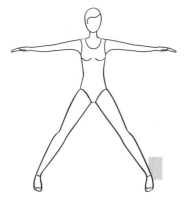
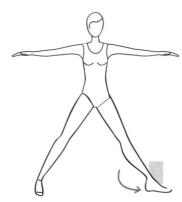
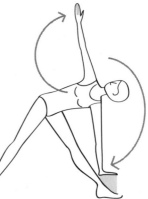

Triangle (page 182)

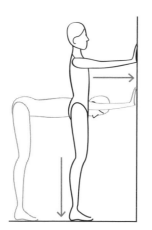
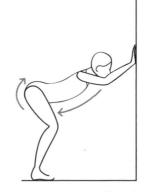
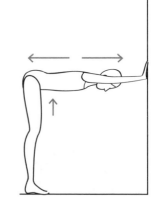

Down Dog at the Wall (page 166)

GAINING STRENGTH
SAMPLE PRACTICE—90 MINUTES

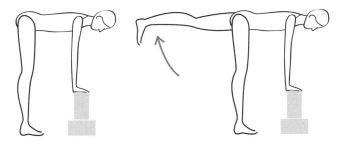

Free Warrior Three (page 188)
(see optional intensification on page 189 if needed)

Slumber Party (page 155)

Part 1, warm up kicks

Part 2, with head turn and foot grab

Butt Kick (page 156)

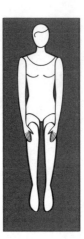 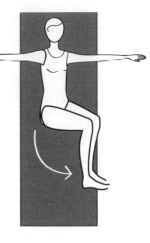

Crunch Twist (page 140)

Part 1,
legs only

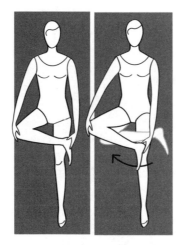 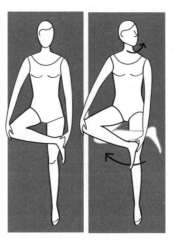

Part 2,
with head turns

Leg Rocking (page 136)

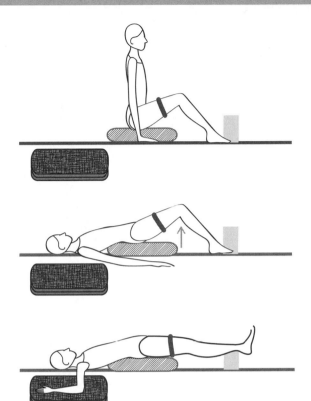

Restorative Shoulderstand (page 190)

Savasana/Sunset Pose (page 197)

*Life is either a daring
adventure
or nothing at all.*

HELEN KELLER

Joanne, cancer survivor

8

Poses to Target
Common Side Effects

As we have discussed, often the side effects of cancer and its treatments can be debilitating and long lasting. Side effects like lymphedema, constipation, weight gain, anxiety, and bone loss need daily management in order to help a survivor feel normal—to perform daily tasks without discomfort or frustration. Other side effects like detoxification after chemotherapy or restriction and discomfort caused by scar tissue require focused support based on an individual's treatments and how the person is feeling and how the body is reacting.

The categorized poses in this chapter are designed to help manage some of the most common side effects. For best results these should be used in conjunction with the complete sequences from chapter 7. This will enable all the benefits of yoga to be fully realized. However, the side effect categories below can be used alone as a focused treatment on a given day.

I have selected poses that I have found to be the most effective for managing each side effect, although there are many others that can also help. My hope is to provide you with as many tools and insights so that you can best manage your own recovery plan.

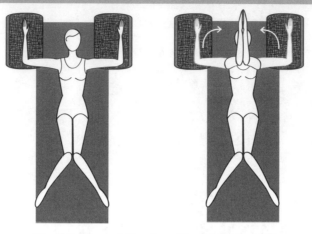

Knock-Kneed Cactus Clap (page 141)

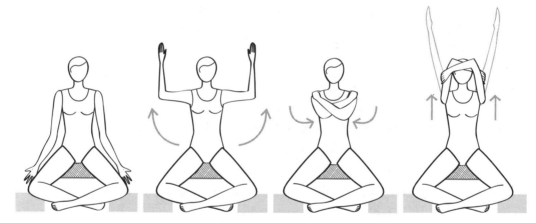

Dirty T-Shirt (page 130)

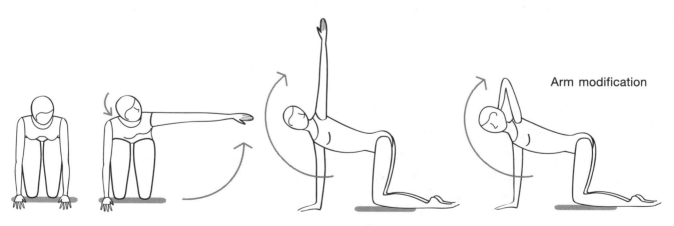

Arm modification

Hands and Knees Twist (page 146)

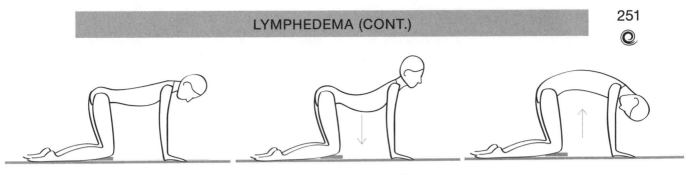

Cat and Cow (page 145)

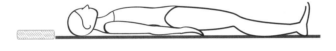

Part 1, just feet

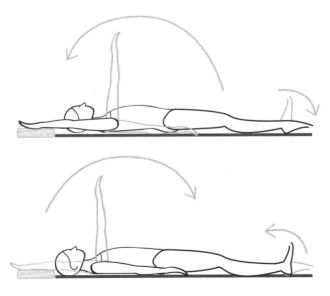

Part 2, with arms

Full-Body Stretch (page 134)

BONE LOSS

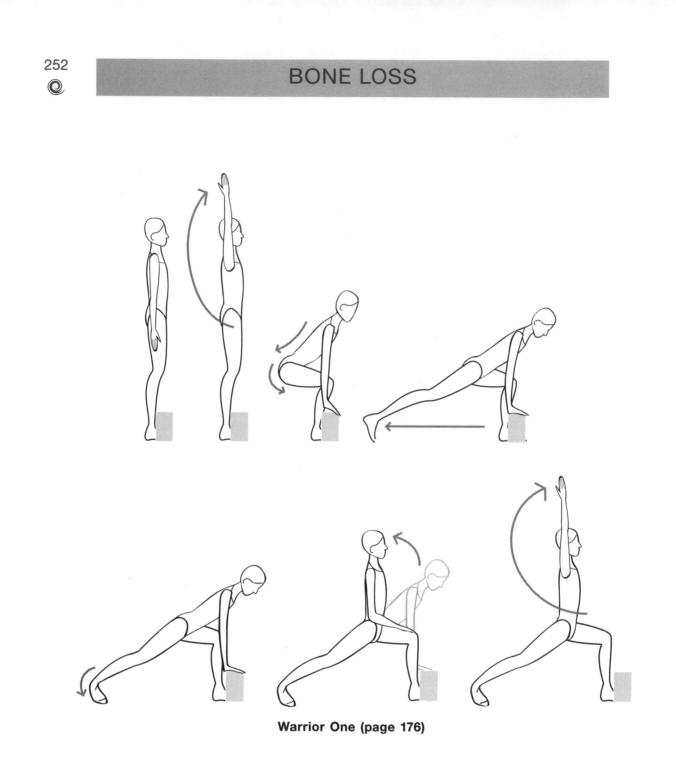

Warrior One (page 176)

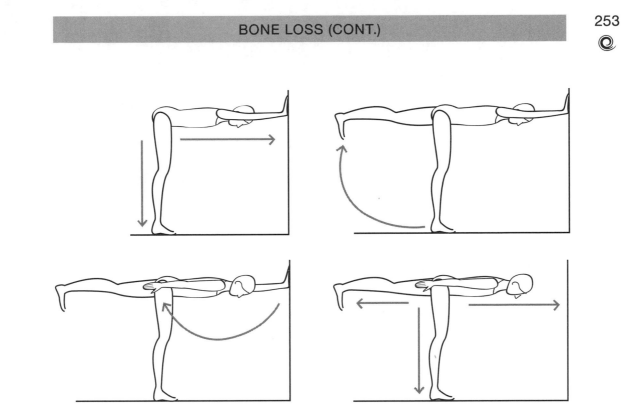

Optional intensification, remove hands from wall

Warrior Three at the Wall (page 186)

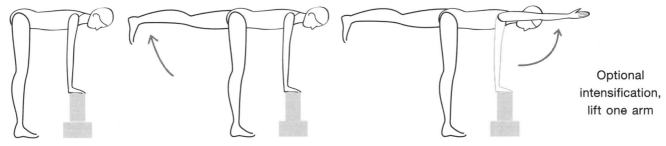

Free Warrior Three (page 188)

Optional
intensification,
lift one arm

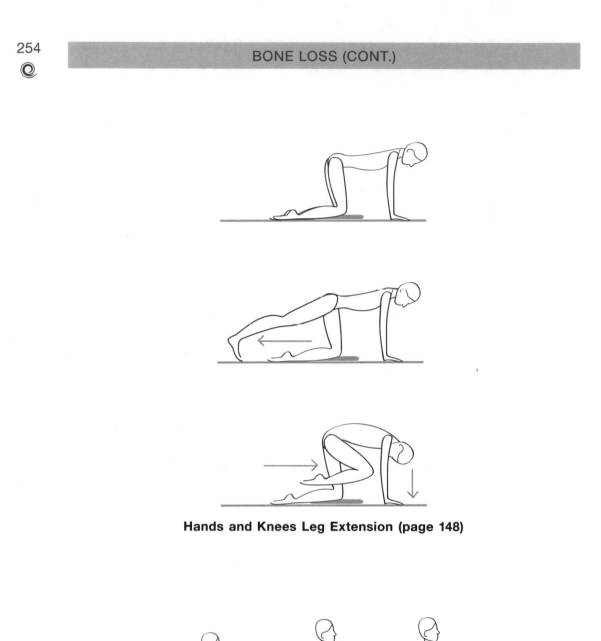

Hands and Knees Leg Extension (page 148)

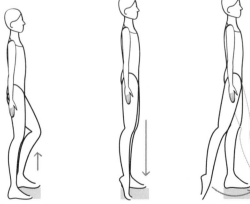

Optional
intensification,
swing foot back
and forth

Stand Tall on One Foot (page 184)

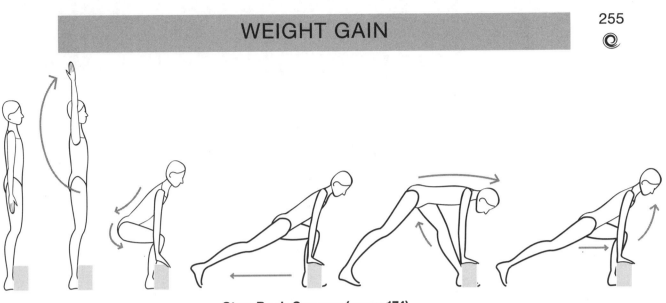

Step Back Seesaw (page 174)

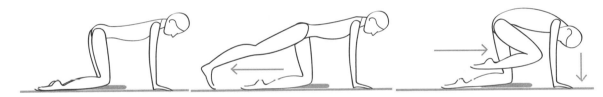

Hands and Knees Leg Extension (page 148)

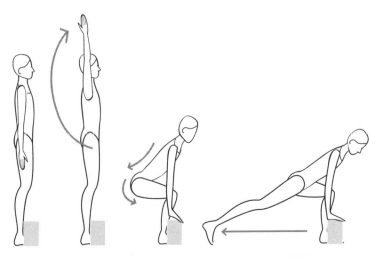

Step Back Sun Salutation (page 168)

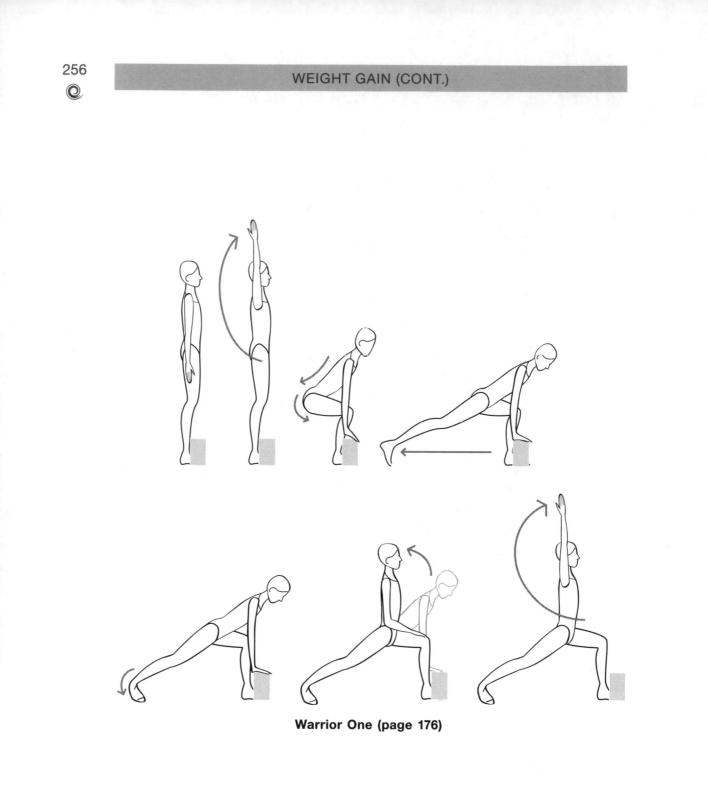

Warrior One (page 176)

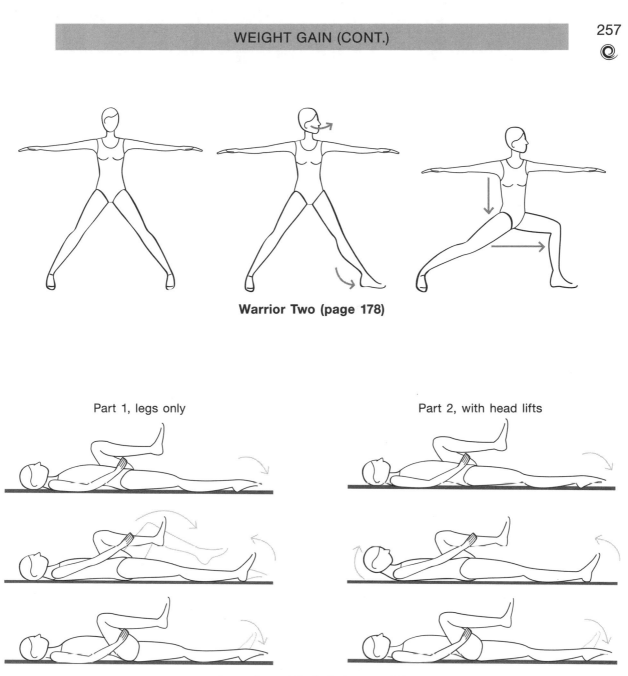

Warrior Two (page 178)

Part 1, legs only

Part 2, with head lifts

Crunch and Switch (page 138)

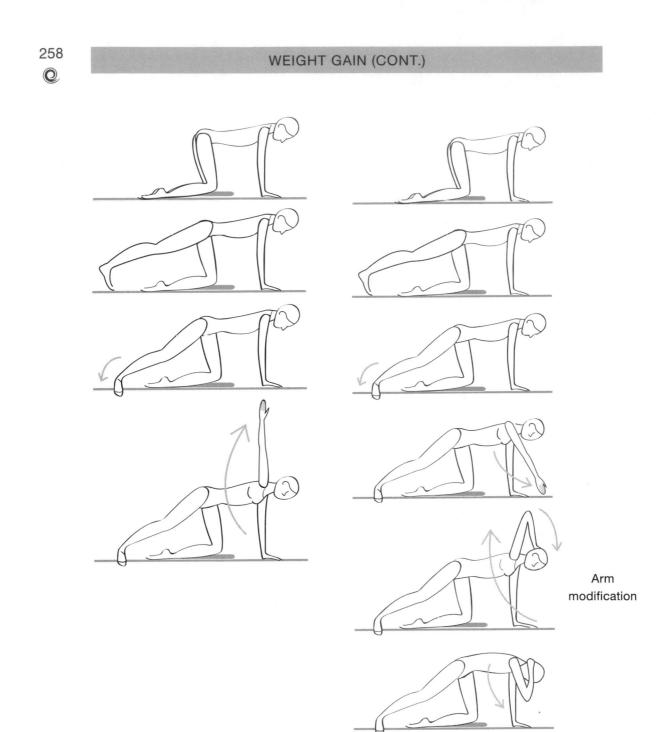

Arm
modification

Twist Extension (page 150)

RANGE OF MOTION/SCAR TISSUE—
UPPER BODY

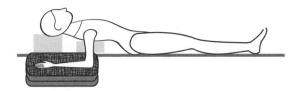

Restorative Fish (page 195)

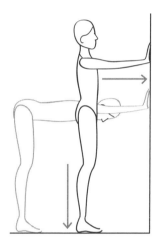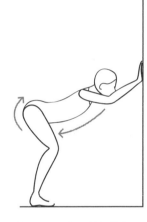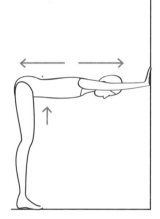

Down Dog at the Wall (page 166)

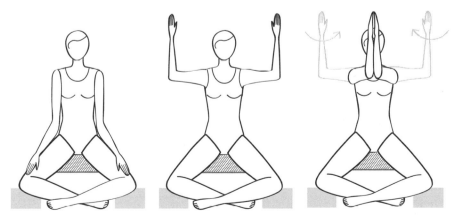

Cactus Clap (page 127)

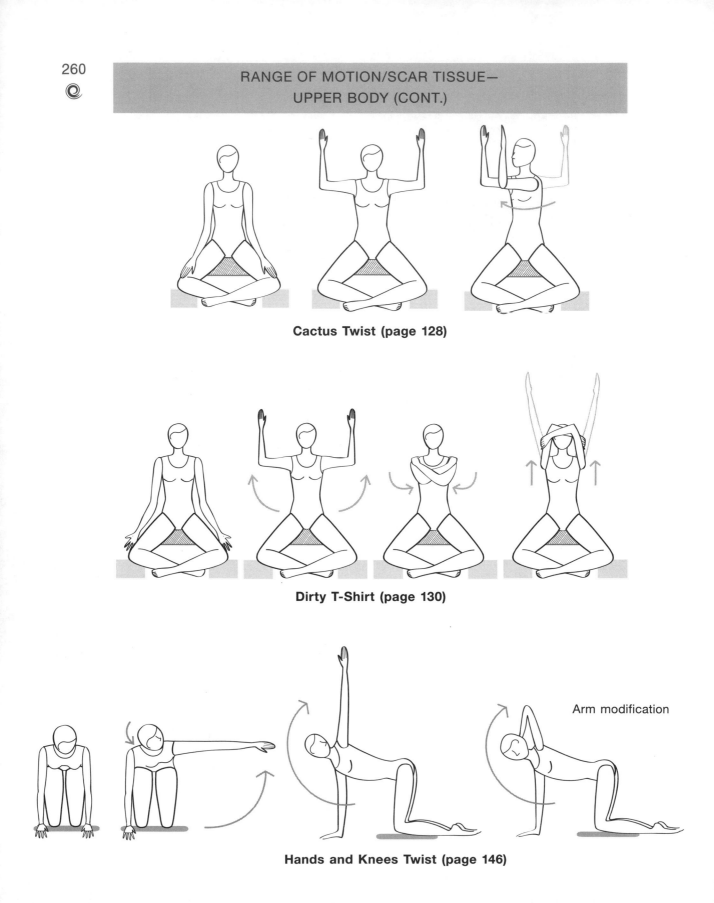

Cactus Twist (page 128)

Dirty T-Shirt (page 130)

Arm modification

Hands and Knees Twist (page 146)

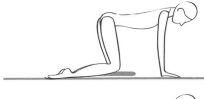

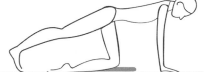

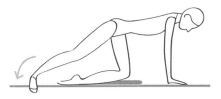

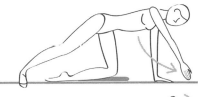

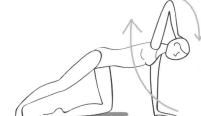

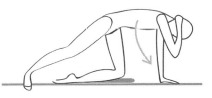

Arm
modification

Twist Extension (page 150)

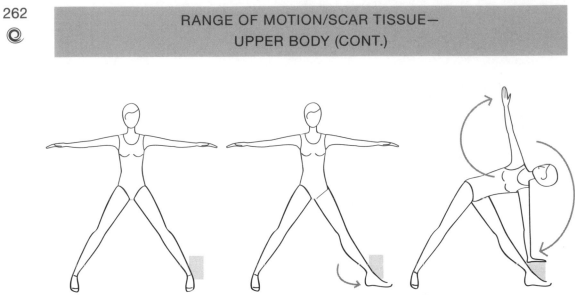

Triangle (page 182)

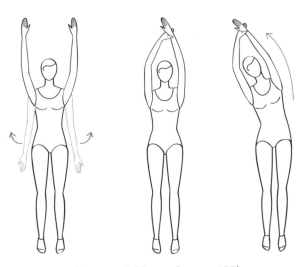

Crescent Moon (page 165)

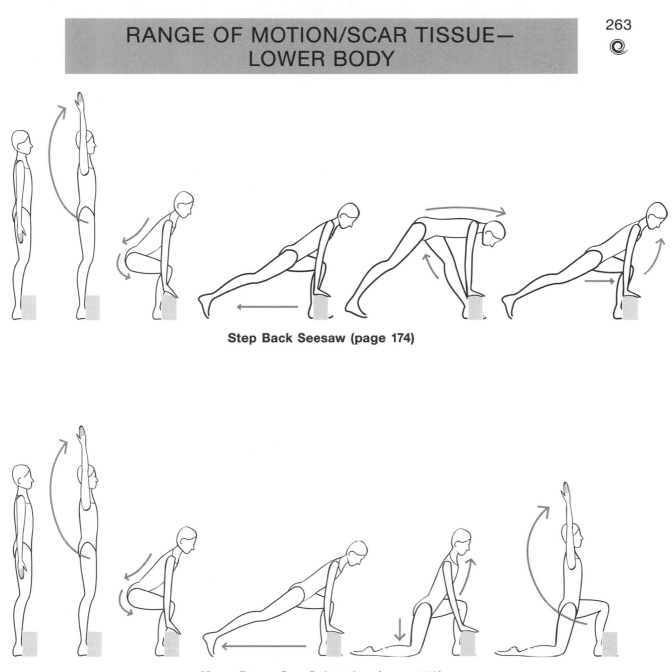

Step Back Seesaw (page 174)

Knee-Down Sun Salutation (page 170)

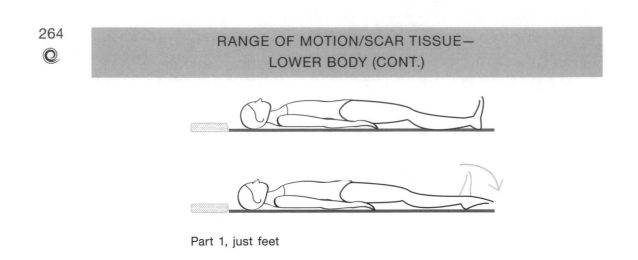

Part 1, just feet

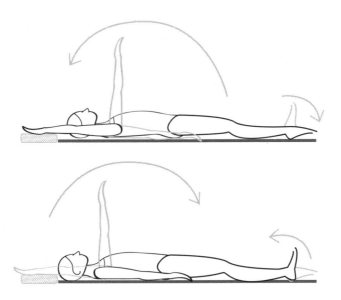

Part 2, with arms

Full-Body Stretch (page 134)

Restorative Fish (page 195)

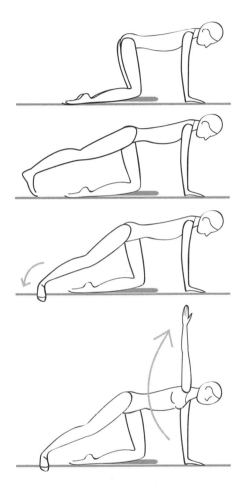

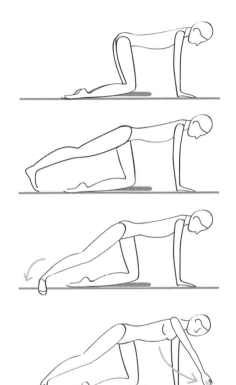

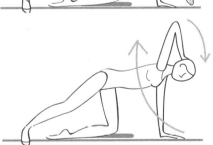

Arm
modification

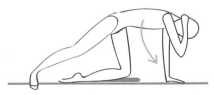

Twist Extension (page 150)

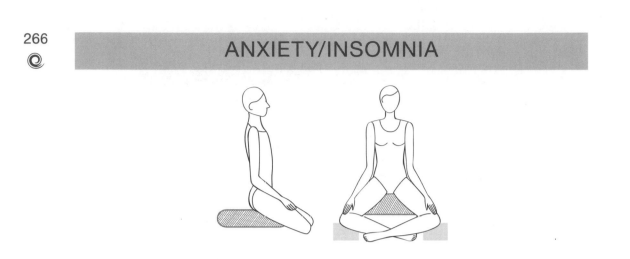

Dynamic Stillness/Breathing/Meditation (pages 115–22)

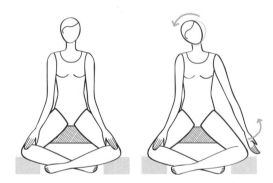

Neck Stretch (page 124)

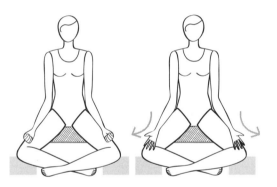

Gather and Hold (page 125)

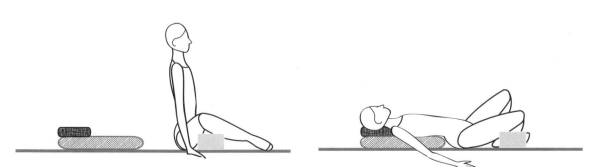

Restorative Cobbler (page 192)

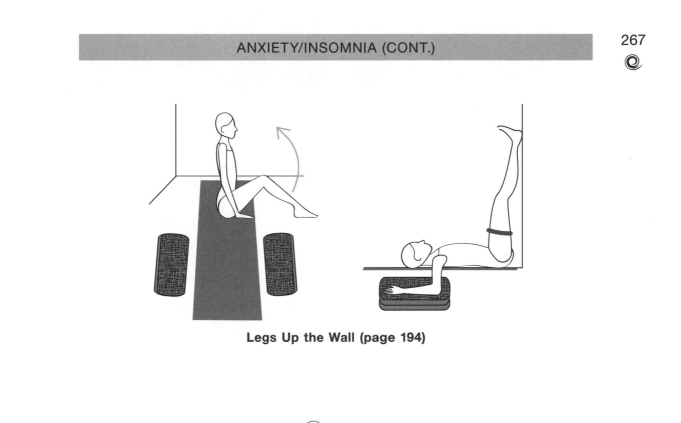

Legs Up the Wall (page 194)

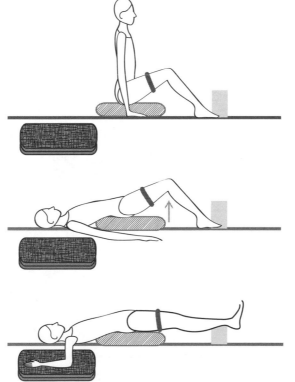

Restorative Shoulderstand (page 190)

CONSTIPATION/BLOATING/ ABDOMINAL OBSTRUCTION

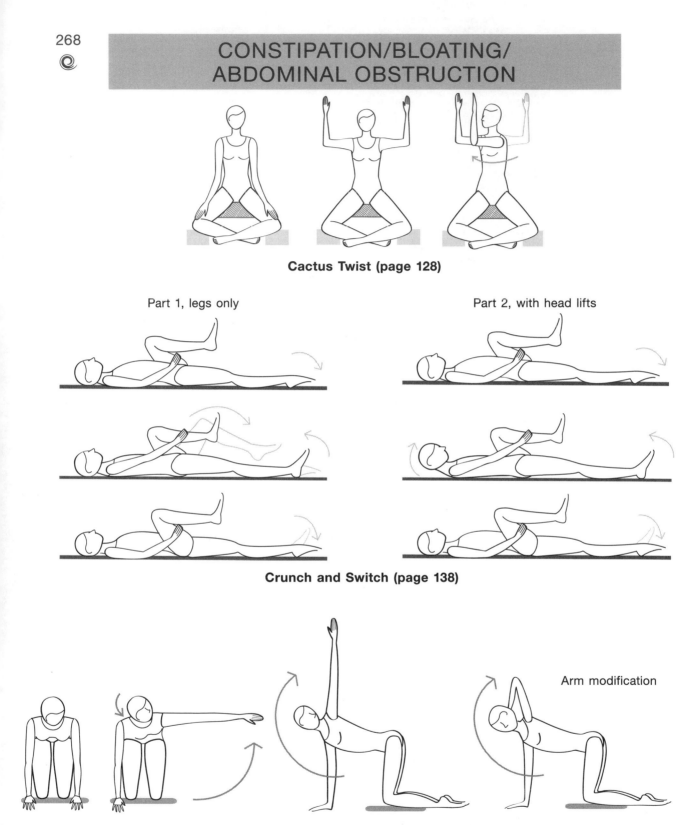

Cactus Twist (page 128)

Part 1, legs only

Part 2, with head lifts

Crunch and Switch (page 138)

Arm modification

Hands and Knees Twist (page 146)

CONSTIPATION/BLOATING/ ABDOMINAL OBSTRUCTION (CONT.)

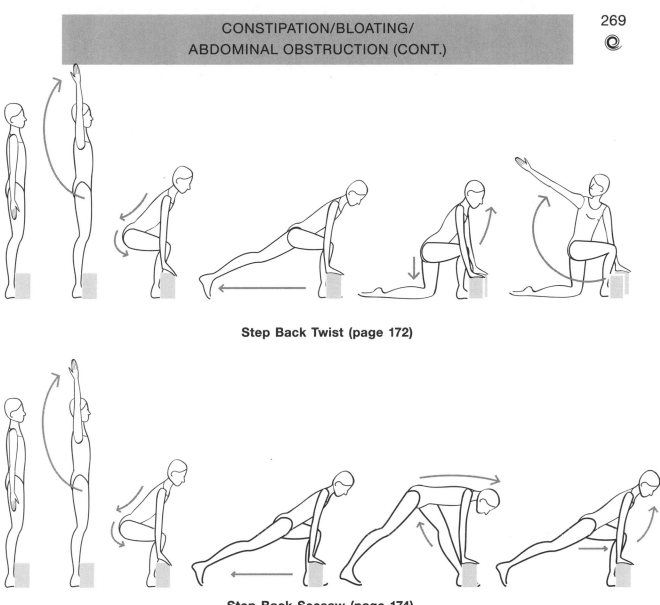

Step Back Twist (page 172)

Step Back Seesaw (page 174)

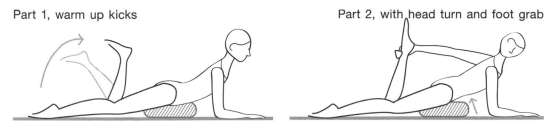

Part 1, warm up kicks

Part 2, with head turn and foot grab

Butt Kick (page 156)

DETOXIFICATION

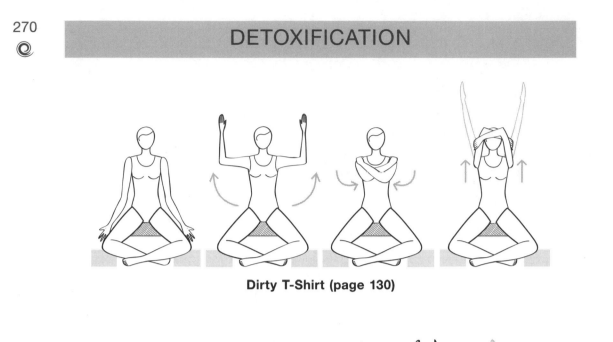

Dirty T-Shirt (page 130)

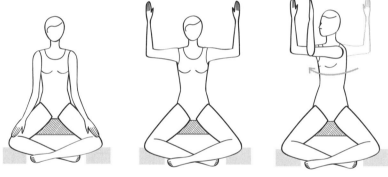

Cactus Twist (page 128)

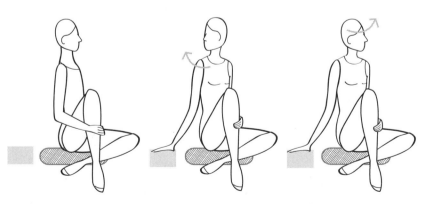

Knee-Up Seated Twist (page 133)

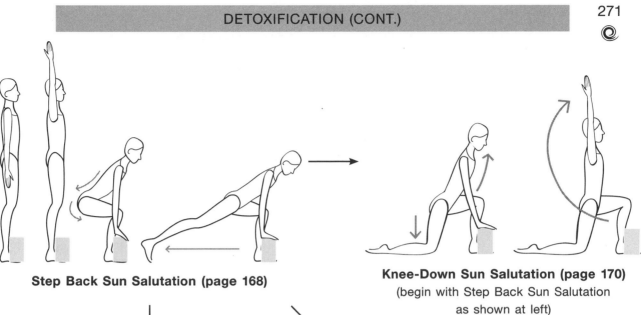

Step Back Sun Salutation (page 168)

Knee-Down Sun Salutation (page 170)
(begin with Step Back Sun Salutation
as shown at left)

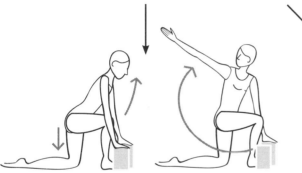

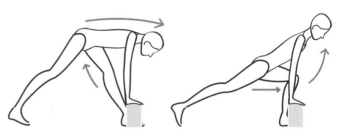

Step Back Twist (page 172)
(begin with Step Back Sun Salutation
as shown above left)

Step Back Seesaw (page 174)
(begin with Step Back Sun Salutation
as shown above left)

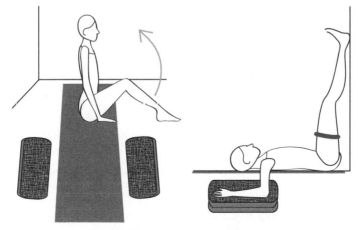

Legs Up the Wall (page 194)

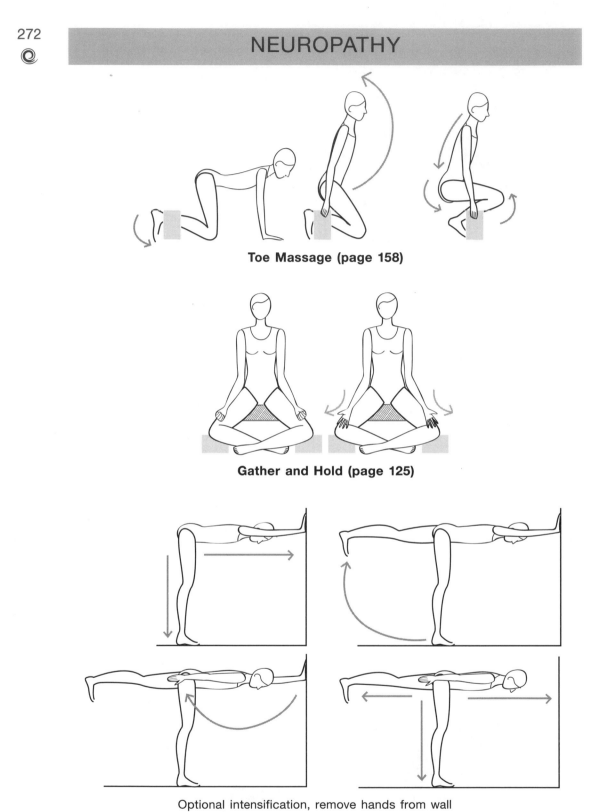

Toe Massage (page 158)

Gather and Hold (page 125)

Optional intensification, remove hands from wall

Warrior Three at the Wall (page 186)

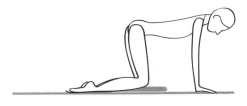
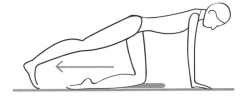
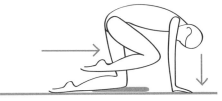

Hands and Knees Leg Extension (page 148)

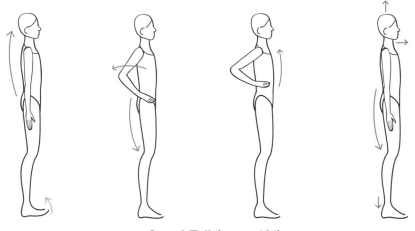

Stand Tall (page 161)

INCONTINENCE

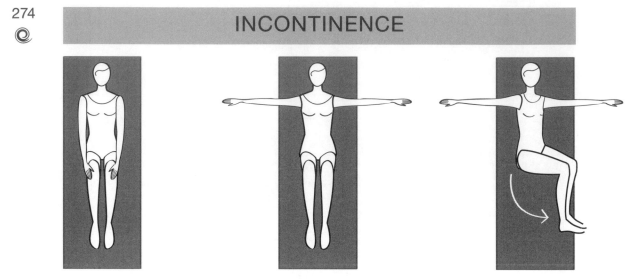

Crunch Twist (page 140)

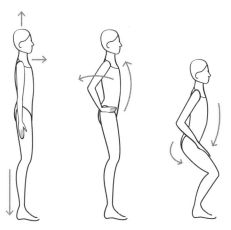

Chair Pose (page 164)

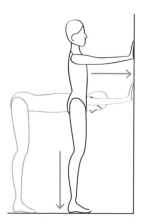
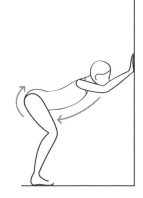
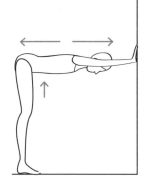

Down Dog at the Wall (page 166)

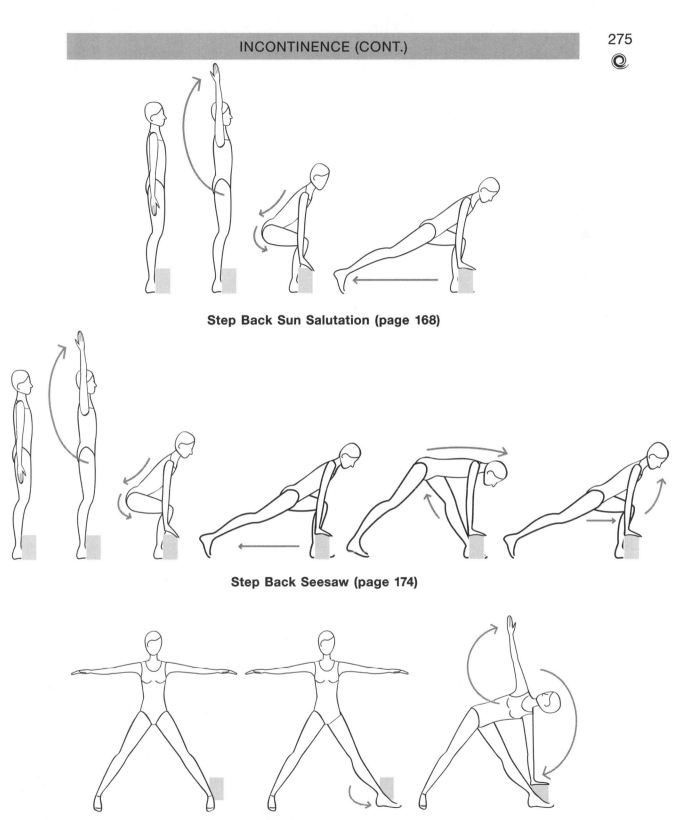

Step Back Sun Salutation (page 168)

Step Back Seesaw (page 174)

Triangle (page 182)

Yoga taught me how to sit with discomfort, not run away from fear, and accept impermanence as the only permanent part of life.

—TARI PRINSTER

Anne and Lina, cancer survivors

Cancer Steals Your Breath, Yoga Gives It Back

Earlier in the book I compared cancer to falling off a swing as a child. It all happens so suddenly, doesn't it—the shock, hitting the hard ground, the sharp pain and embarrassment in front of friends leading to tears. That was my experience many years ago when first hearing my doctor say, "You have cancer." As we grow older, swings become bicycles, relationships, or a problem at work. We fall off, get hurt, and we get back up.

Bringing this book to a close, I invite you to think about change, all kinds of change. Cancer is a special life challenge, to be sure. But it is not the only one we have had in life, and it is very likely not the last. "There is nothing permanent except change," said Greek philosopher Heraclitus of Ephesus. Best to be prepared for new surprises—some lovely, others that frighten.

Cancer cells change and adapt to treatments like chemotherapy. So, too, is our understanding of cancer changing, along with our understanding of the best treatments and ways to cope. Today we learn that effective treatment requires personalized solutions for each survivor, often at the molecular-genetic level. A hundred years from now I believe people will look back on current theory about cancer and treatments like chemotherapy or radiation as primitive, blunt tools. They are like the practice of bloodletting in the nineteenth century that today seems crude. These medical procedures may be the best we have, but they are not the targeted, individualized intervention that a molecular disorder demands.

Cancer is a fact of life, especially now that many people in the West are living longer. One in three people will have some form of cancer in their lifetime; of that number, one in four will eventually die from it. So cancer is not a death sentence—it should be treated as a manageable disease. Of course, no one can totally control the path of all complex cancers, but we are neither helpless nor without resources. Human beings have this remarkable capacity, which has evolved over hundreds of thousands of years, to adapt to nearly any environment or any of life's challenges, however bad.

I'll share a small story. Just after I got my diagnosis in 2000, my younger sister sent me a small stone to hold and rub when times got rough. More spiritual than I was at the time, my sister called it a goddess stone. I was to use it to guide reflection and to calm myself during anxious moments. I have reached for it often in my pocket and used it well in the years since my diagnosis. Indeed, this small stone gave me pause to reflect. Today, I share these reflections in my classes and leave them with you. Take the ideas in this book with you wherever you go. When something happens you don't expect, you can use them for reflection and inspiration, to improve the quality of your life, and for those moments in life when new challenges appear, as they surely will.

As survivors we seek a flexible stance in life so that when we fall or get hurt, we absorb the shock, dust ourselves off, and get back on the swing. Yes, it's easier said than done. But below are several related ideas to keep in mind as you move—nimble and ever hopeful—through recovery to new challenges. These are "five pearls of wisdom"—influenced by ancient concepts in Buddhism and other spiritual traditions. Think of these as guiding ideas for a spiritual practice to prepare your mind and emotions for whatever life brings, good and not so good.

 Challenges are gifts that force us to search for a new center of gravity. Don't fight them. Just find a new way to stand.
OPRAH WINFREY

1. You've got the power. So much of getting cancer is about losing control: control of your body, your emotions, your bowels, and even temperature regulation in your body. You lose control of your job, your place in relationships, your finances, and even what you wear. Doctors and therapists offer help, but they are now in control, not you. Understandably, we give control to specialists in the hope they will "cure" us. Friends and even strangers offer their advice, sometimes without asking what you want or think.

At the same time, massive energy has to go into making difficult decisions about which doctor to see, what kind of treatment is necessary and with which side effects, or for how long. What does this test result mean? Are there better treatments I can find on the web? Should I get another opinion? How much will it cost and am I covered by insurance? The steady march of critical decisions is without end and it is exhausting.

All this change can be overwhelming, making it difficult for a person to know what she feels and wants. Overloaded by clinical options and friendly advice, the survivor learns to listen to her own mind and body. What are *you* feeling? We learn practical tools like meditation to begin to take back our life. To rebuild a sense of control so that it's even better than before cancer is neither simple nor fast. A daily yoga practice can help.

The sacred writings of Hindu, Buddhist, and yogic traditions include ethical guidelines and rules of behavior designed to support us on life's path. I like to think of them as the reins we can take hold of literally and figuratively. For example, in yogic philosophy there are ethical and spiritual precepts called *yamas* and *niyamas*. The first yama is *ahimsa*—nonviolence. Or, in other words, act with kindness. Starting with yourself, of course. Be gentle. An act of self-loving kindness can be as simple as slowing your breathing or sitting up straight. Just doing that much yoga can give you the control of the reins you may need when things seem to be falling apart.

2. No identity crisis. A difficult part of getting cancer that is not often written or talked about is that it can temporarily steal your sense of self. You think if only you had not smoked, had gone on that diet, eaten more tofu, or not stood so close to the microwave. Perhaps you would not be sick if you had only managed stress better. Or perhaps you feel that earlier in life you had done something wrong and are now suffering for your mistake. These feelings of being so conspicuous, of having made a bad mistake, and that family and friends, even strangers may see us as "not normal" make us uncomfortable, deeply so. Such feelings are irrational, but saying that doesn't make them go away.

Personally, I live with these questions and doubts. But I know that the search for the "one cause" is futile and a distraction from the hard work of managing the cancer (rather than it managing me). To wonder what, years ago, I could have done differently is irrational because most cancers have many, many hidden causes, most well outside personal control. Better to think of cancer as a mystery because no one can say exactly what caused your type of cell mutation, or why the immune system did not catch that first mutating cell. The true causes will always remain a secret. Can we live with that explanation?

Perhaps we feel exposed—even shy—in front of friends and family. Worse, some of my students say they even feel guilty, as if they have done something wrong.

No one likes to feel conspicuous, vulnerable, or guilty. No one wants to appear weak, frail, and sick. What survivors want most is to feel normal—and that is how we want others to treat us.

I ask survivors to recognize these intruding thoughts and feelings, even if they are understandable human reactions. Most importantly, you can learn to say: "I'm okay, I'm me. This is who I am and this is what I want." In doing so, you take up your personal space in a vast universe just like everyone else. You don't have to apologize for anything.

3. Sit a while. Learn to sit with discomfort—a challenge, I know. Buddhists believe that human suffering is caused by the attachments people have to ideas and things—pleasant or unpleasant—and they ask us to step back a pace or two. There is a valuable lesson in taking a pause. The ideas or sensations that crowd the mind can be so seductive. Yes, I want to live, I want to be without fears, I want to be healthy; no, I don't want to die or feel sick. Most of all, I want to feel normal. I want my breast back, I want to breathe easily. Hey, what I really want is to be like I was before cancer!

Each of these desires, or attachments, is understandable, especially when we are battling a serious disease—but, if we let the mind dwell on them, we suffer even more. We want to recognize these ideas and feelings as psychological attachments that can be managed, however persistent or intrusive in daily consciousness.

Learn to recognize each idea or sensation, but hold each one at arm's length and pause. Try not to respond to feelings, ideas, or sensations—just look at them as uninvited guests. Work hard to not let mental desires control consciousness and thus daily existence. By doing so, we learn to accept life here and now rather than live too much in the past or future. We begin to move toward a new normal and this is the beginning of the healing.

I believe we can get most of our needs met if we declare what we need and truly want. Yoga can help us live with whatever challenge cancer brings, including dying. Call it "sitting well with discomfort" rather than denying or dwelling on it. Just sit a while.

4. Turn off the chatter. Yoga teaches us how to do this by increasing awareness of body sensations as well as the ebb and flow of daily consciousness. Yoga teaches us to listen, really listen, to the body and its sensations as well as to the mind and its steady stream of ideas and emotions.

We do yoga for insight into how the body works. We use yoga to help us turn off the monkey mind in order to hear what's really going on.

We listen to our breathing and develop new confidence in our minds and bodies, perhaps a new spiritual side of ourselves. In so doing, we are made stronger by having a body that is supple, rested, and well managed. Rather than let ourselves be flooded with negative ideas and frightening thoughts, we learn to manage consciousness, which helps us cope with cancer and treatments—and the rest of life. None of this is easy, but this practice gives us the basic tools to live a mindful life—full of joy, wonder, and hope.

5. Live in the Now. Instead of living with disappointments, which will be endless, we live in the Now, this fleeting moment, this very second that we are alive.

Below is a traditional Buddhist story I like. I hope it will inspire survivors everywhere to continue seeking and creating happiness, love, and health.

Every morning a Buddhist nun walked through the forest. One clear, crisp morning, she heard a rustling in the leaves and looked up to see a large tiger watching her from a distance. Sensing that the tiger was about to attack, she started running as fast as she could, only to come to a clearing leading to a steep cliff. Not seeing any other way to go, the nun grasped a large vine running partly down the cliff's side, and began to climb down just as the tiger arrived. So there she was, hanging, grasping the narrow end of a vine, with a snarling tiger above her and a deep canyon beneath her. To make matters worse, a mouse appeared and began to gnaw on the vine just above her, but out of reach. Just then, the nun noticed a wild strawberry plant growing from the side of the cliff, with one plump red strawberry. She reached out, picked the berry, put it in her mouth, and thought to herself, "This strawberry is delicious!"

Going forward, I invite you to taste the sweet strawberry that is within your reach, forgetting the tiger and the mouse. Find time for yourself through yoga or any other practice of self-healing. Create space in life to take in the simple small things like sitting quietly before a window in winter, watching the gentle snow fall.

Namaste.

Life is an opportunity, benefit from it.

Life is beauty, admire it.

Life is a dream, realize it.

Life is a challenge, meet it.

Life is a duty, complete it.

Life is a game, play it.

Life is a promise, fulfill it.

Life is sorrow, overcome it.

Life is a song, sing it.

Life is a struggle, accept it.

Life is a tragedy, confront it.

Life is an adventure, dare it.

Life is luck, make it.

Life is too precious, do not destroy it.

Life is life, fight for it.

UNKOWN POET

Resources for Survivors, Teachers, and Caretakers

Research and resources on both cancer and yoga are constantly evolving, with both fields still in their infancy. So I encourage my students, both survivors and yoga practitioners, to embrace the curiosity that leads you to read this book. Continuously learn the facts, dispel myths, and gain knowledge to be truly compassionate to yourself or others.

To provide a comprehensive or timeless resource list would be impossible as research is actively being conducted and new findings identified on both cancer and yoga. So I am going to provide you a list of resources that I used to develop this book and my methodology and which I consult daily. This is not an exhaustive list but I hope it provides fuel for your curiosity.

One quick piece of advice. In my journey I have encountered articles, research findings, and studies that were outstanding and intriguing. And potentially these could have led me down other paths. If I had not dug further into who was paying for the research or interrogated the hypothesis with an eye for fact-based information, I could have easily been mislead. I strongly urge you to use your curiosity to interrogate everything you read and find. Use the resources below to verify or challenge any learnings.

CANCER RESOURCES AND SUPPORT INFORMATION

American Cancer Society: cancer.org
National Cancer Institute: cancer.gov

Cancer Research UK: cancerresearchuk.org

US National Library of Medicine: PubMed.gov—The ultimate resource for the latest scientific fact-based research

Breast Cancer Action: bcaction.org—Offers information, webinars, tools, and movements to end the breast cancer epidemic and improve the lives of those fighting it

Breastcancer.org—Latest research information, very helpful webinars, podcasts, and other resources

National Lymphedema Network: lymphnet.org—Provides research, resources, support groups, and a network of professional massage and lymphedema specialists

Cure Magazine: curetoday.com—Interprets research and latest findings in a thoughtful and pragmatic way; easier to read!

CANCER ADVOCACY ORGANIZATIONS

Young Survival Coalition: youngsurvival.org—Resource and advocacy for young women facing breast cancer

Patient Advocate Foundation: patientadvocate.org—Resource and advocacy for insurance and health care access problems

4wholeness.com—Resource and advocacy for overall well-being for women with or recovering from breast cancer

Health Monitor: healthmonitor.com—Resource and advocacy for achieving and monitoring healthy life choices, especially for those suffering from cancer or other illnesses

YOGA REFERENCES
AND PUBLICATIONS

International Association of Yoga Therapists (IAYT): iayt.org—Yoga therapy works to bridge the gap between yoga and health care

Sciatica.org—Research findings and news about yoga, osteoporosis, and other topics

Lilias! Yoga Gets Better With Age, Lilias Folan, Rodale, 2005

OM Yoga: A Guide to Daily Practice, Cyndi Lee, Chronicle Books, 2002

Science of Breath: A Practical Guide, Swami Rama, Rudolph Ballentine, M.D., Alan Hymes, M.D., The Himalayan Institute Press, 1979

The Breathing Book, Donna Farhi, Owl Books, Henry Holt & Co., 1996

The Woman's Book of Yoga & Health, Linda Sparrowe, Shambhala
Publications, 2002

Yoga for Wellness, Gary Kraftsow, Penguin Compass,1999

30 Essential Yoga Poses: For Beginning Students and Their Teachers,
Judith Lasater, Ph.D., P.T., Rodmell Press, 2003

ABOUT YOGA4CANCER

For more information about the y4c methodology, classes, trainings, research,
and events visit y4c.com. Other useful y4c resources include:

y4c Trained Teachers: Not all yoga or yoga teachers are the same. Working
with the cancer community requires facts, understanding, and experience
of the physical and emotional impacts of cancer and its treatment. For a
list of y4c trained teachers in your area, please go to y4c.com.

y4c on Facebook: Found under Yoga 4 Cancer. To get the latest information on the intersection of yoga and cancer, join in our community. We
are dedicated to providing the latest research, insights, and information
to our community of cancer survivors and yoga practitioners.

Notes

2. THE SCIENCE OF CANCER AND YOGA

1. American Cancer Society, "Cancer Treatment and Survivorship Facts and Figures 2012–2013," 1.

2. Kirkwood, et al. "Yoga for Anxiety," bjsm.bmj.com/content/39/12/884.full; and "Yoga for Anxiety and Depression," www.health.harvard.edu/newsletters/Harvard_Mental_Health_Letter/2009/April/Yoga-for-anxiety-and-depression.

3. Anderson, et al. "Breathing Variability," www.ncbi.nlm.nih.gov/pmc/articles/PMC2752321.

4. American Cancer Society, "Physical Activity and the Cancer Patient," www.cancer.org/treatment/survivorshipduringandaftertreatment/stayingactive/physical-activity-and-the-cancer-patient.

5. Ornish, *The Spectrum*.

6. Rockhill et al., "Physical Activity and Mortality," www.ncbi.nlm.nih.gov/pmc/articles/PMC1446638/pdf/11291369.pdf. For an exhaustive treatment of the benefits of exercise on health outcomes from the American Heart Association, see also Kokkinos and Myers, "Exercise and Physical Activity."

7. Holmes et al., "Physical Activity and Survival," jama.jamanetwork.com/article.aspx?articleid=200955.

8. Blech, *Healing through Exercise*.

9. Sharma and Haider, "Yoga as an Alternative and Complementary Treatment."

10. Kushi et al., "American Cancer Society Guidelines," http://onlinelibrary.wiley.com/doi/10.3322/caac.20140/full.

11. Singh et al., "Physical Activity and Performance," 49, http://archpedi.jamanetwork.com/article.aspx?articleid=1107683.

12. Iyengar, *Light on Yoga*.

13. Benson, *The Relaxation Response*.

14. Ader and Cohen, "Behaviorally Conditioned Immunosuppression."

15. American Cancer Society, "Attitudes and Cancer," www.cancer.org/treatment/ treatmentsandsideeffects/emotionalsideeffects/attitudes-and-cancer.

16. Kytle, *To Want to Learn,* 104.

17. For a recent overview and positive "vision" of CAM, see Barnett and Shale, "The Integration of Complementary and Alternative Medicine."

18. Hildebrand et al., "Recreational Physical Activity."

3. APPLYING THE SCIENCE
FOR RECOVERY AND PREVENTION

1. "Yoga in America Study 2012," www.yogajournal.com/press/yoga_in_america.

2. Schaffer, "Do Our Bones Influence Our Minds?," www.newyorker.com/online/ blogs/elements/2013/11/do-our-bones-influence-our-minds.html.

3. "Bone Health," www.macmillan.org.uk/Cancerinformation/Livingwithandaftercancer/ Lifeaftercancer/Bonehealth.aspx.

4. Yung et al., "Effects of Weight Bearing," bjsm.bmj.com/content/39/8/547.long.

5. Fishman, "Yoga for Osteoporosis," www.sciatica.org/downloads/YogaOsteoporosis_ PilotStudy.pdf.

6. Satin, Linden, and Millman, "Yoga and Psychophysiological Determinants."

7. Fishman, "Private Study and New Book," www.huffingtonpost.com/loren-fishman-md/pilot-study-and-new-book_b_384430.html.

8. Smith and Boser, "Yoga, Vertebral Fractures, and Osteoporosis: Research and Recommendations," www.undulationexercise.com/publications/yoga-vertebral-fractures-and-osteoporosis.pdf.

9. American Cancer Society, www.cancer.org.

10. Qu et al., "Rapid Gene Expression," www.plosone.org/article/info%3Adoi%2F10.1371 %2Fjournal.pone.0061910.

11. Mandal, "What Is Gene Expression?" www.news-medical.net/health/What-is-Gene-Expression.aspx.

12. American Cancer Society, www.cancer.org.

13. Dhananjai et al., "Reducing Psychological Distress," www.ncbi.nlm.nih.gov/pmc/ articles/PMC3573546.

14. Buffart et al., "Physical and Psychosocial Benefits of Yoga," www.biomedcentral. com/1471-2407/12/559.

15. Mackenzie et al., "Affect and Mindfulness," www.ncbi.nlm.nih.gov/pmc/articles/ PMC3676912.

16. Streeter et al., "Effects of Yoga," online.liebertpub.com/doi/pdf/10.1089/ acm.2010.0007.

17. Mustian et al., "Multicenter, Randomized Controlled Trial of Yoga for Sleep Quality Among Cancer Survivors."

18. Sephton et al., "Depression, Cortisol, and Suppressed Cell-Mediated Immunity in Metastatic Breast Cancer."

19. Novotney, "Yoga as a Practice Tool," www.apa.org/monitor/2009/11/yoga.aspx.

20. Costanzo, Ryff, and Singer, "Psychosocial Adjustment Among Cancer Survivors," www.ncbi.nlm.nih.gov/pmc/articles/PMC2668871.

21. Quoted in Wiley-Blackwell, "Yoga Provides Emotional Benefits," www.sciencedaily .com/releases/2009/02/090224230707.htm.

4. THE Y4C METHODOLOGY

1. Goodwin et al., "The Effect of Group Psychosocial Support," www.nejm.org/doi/full/10.1056/NEJMoa011871#t=articleTop.

2. Rama, *Meditation and Its Practice*.

3. Carlson and Garland, "Impact of Mindfulness-Based Stress Reduction."

4. Iyengar, *Light on Life*, 28.

Bibliography

Ader, Robert, and Nicholas Cohen. "Behaviorally Conditioned Immunosuppression." *Psychosomatic Medicine* 37, no. 4 (1975): 333–40.

American Cancer Society. "Attitudes and Cancer." March 31, 2014. www.cancer.org/treatment/treatmentsandsideeffects/emotionalsideeffects/attitudes-and-cancer.

———. "Cancer Treatment and Survivorship Facts and Figures 2012–2013." Atlanta, Ga.: American Cancer Society, 2012. www.cancer.org/acs/groups/content/@epidemiologysurveilance/documents/document/acspc-033876.pdf.

———. *Lymphedema: Understanding and Managing Lymphedema After Cancer Treatment.* Atlanta, Ga.: American Cancer Society, 2006.

———. "Physical Activity and the Cancer Patient." February 06, 2013. www.cancer.org/treatment/survivorshipduringandaftertreatment/stayingactive/physical-activity-and-the-cancer-patient.

Anderson, David E., Jessica D. McNeely, Margaret A. Chesney, and Beverly G. Windham. "Breathing Variability at Rest Is Positively Associated with 24-Hr Blood Pressure Level." *American Journal of Hypertension* 21, no. 12 (2008): 1324–29. www.ncbi.nlm.nih.gov/pmc/articles/PMC2752321.

Barnett, Jeffrey E., and Allison J. Shale. "The Integration of Complementary and Alternative Medicine (CAM) Into the Practice of Psychology: A Vision for the Future." *Professional Psychology: Research and Practice* 43, no. 6 (2012): 576–85.

Benson, Herbert. *The Relaxation Response.* Revised edition. New York: Avon Books, 2000. First published 1976.

Blech, Jörg. *Healing through Exercise: Scientifically-Proven Ways to Prevent and Overcome Illness and Lengthen Your Life.* New York: Merloyd Lawrence Books/Perseus, 2009.

Block, Keith I. *Life Over Cancer: The Block Center Program for Integrative Cancer Treatment.* New York: Bantam Books, 2009.

"Bone Health." Macmillan Cancer Support. July 1, 2011. www.macmillan.org.uk/Cancerinformation/Livingwithandaftercancer/Lifeaftercancer/Bonehealth.aspx.

Broad, William J. *The Science of Yoga: The Risks and Rewards.* New York: Simon & Schuster, 2012.

Buffart, Laurien M., Jannique GZ van Uffelen, Ingrid I. Riphagen, Johannes Brug, Willem van Mechelen, Wendy J. Brown, and Mai JM Chinapaw. "Physical and Psychosocial Benefits of Yoga in Cancer Patients and Survivors, a Systematic Review and Meta-Analysis of Randomized Controlled Trials." *BMC Cancer* 12 (2012): 559. www.biomedcentral.com/1471-2407/12/559.

Carlson, Linda E., and Sheila N. Garland. "Impact of Mindfulness-Based Stress Reduction (MSBR) on Sleep, Mood, Stress, and Fatigue Symptoms in Cancer Outpatients." *International Journal of Behavioral Medicine* 12, no. 4 (December 2005): 278–85

Chödrön, Pema. *When Things Fall Apart.* Boston: Shambhala Publications, 1997.

———. *The Pocket Pema Chödrön.* Boston: Shambhala Publications, 2008.

Cohen, Darlene. *Turning Suffering Inside Out: A Zen Approach to Physical and Emotional Pain.* Boston: Shambhala Publications, 2000.

Costanzo, Erin, Carol Ryff, and Burton Singer. "Psychosocial Adjustment among Cancer Survivors: Findings from a National Survey of Health and Well-Being." *Health Psychology* 28 (March 2009): 147–56. www.ncbi.nlm.nih.gov/pmc/articles/PMC2668871.

Coulter, H. David. *Anatomy of Hatha Yoga.* Marlboro, Vt.: Body and Breath, 2002.

Wiley-Blackwell. "Yoga Provides Emotional Benefits to Women with Breast Cancer." *Science Daily* (March 2, 2009). www.sciencedaily.com/releases/2009/02/090224230707.htm.

Dhananjai, S., Sadashiv, Sunita Tiwari, Krishna Dutt, and Rajjan Kumar. "Reducing Psychological Distress and Obesity through Yoga Practice." *International Journal of Yoga Therapy* 6, no. 1 (January–June 2013): 66–70. www.ncbi.nlm.nih.gov/pmc/articles/PMC3573546.

Ehrenreich, Barbara. *Bright-Sided: How Positive Thinking Is Undermining America.* New York: Metropolitan Books, 2009.

Fishman, Loren. "Private Study and New Book Prove Yoga's Benefits in Treating Osteoporosis." *The Huffington Post*, December 8, 2009. www.huffingtonpost.com/loren-fishman-md/pilot-study-and-new-book_b_384430.html.

———. "Yoga for Osteoporosis: A Pilot Study." *Topics in Geriatric Rehabilitation* 25, no. 3 (July/September 2009): 244–50. www.sciatica.org/downloads/YogaOsteoporosis_PilotStudy.pdf.

Foldi, Michael, and Roman Strossenreuther. *Foundations of Manual Lymph Drainage.* Third edition. New York: Elsevier Mosby Press, 2005.

Garcia, Megan. *Mega Yoga: The First Yoga Program for Curvy Women.* New York: DK Publishing, 2006.

Goodwin, Pamela J., Molyn Leszcz, Marguerite Ennis, Jan Koopmans, Leslie Vincent, Helaine Guther, Elaine Drysdale, et al. "The Effect of Group Psychosocial Support on Survival in Metastatic Breast Cancer." *New England Journal of Medicine* 345 (2001): 1719–26. www.nejm.org/doi/full/10.1056/NEJMoa011871#t=article.

Groopman, Jerome. *The Anatomy of Hope: How People Prevail in the Face of Illness*. New York: Random House, 2004.

Hanh, Thich Nhat. *The Miracle of Mindfulness: An Introduction to the Practice of Meditation*. Boston: Beacon Press, 1987.

Harrington, Anne. *The Cure Within: A History of Mind-Body Medicine*. New York: W.W. Norton, 2008.

Harrison, Eric. *How Meditation Heals: Scientific Evidence and Practical Applications*. Berkeley, Calif.: Ulysses Press, 2000.

Harvard Health Publications. "Yoga for Anxiety and Depression." www.health .harvard.edu/newsletters/Harvard_Mental_Health_Letter/2009/April/ Yoga-for-anxiety-and-depression.

Hildebrand, Janet S., Susan M. Gapstur, Peter T. Campbell, Mia M. Gaudet, and Alpa V. Patel. "Recreational Physical Activity and Leisure-Time Sitting in Relation to Postmenopausal Breast Cancer Risk." *Cancer Epidemiology, Biomarkers and Prevention* 22 (October 2013): 1906–12.

Hitchens, Christopher. "Topic of Cancer." *Vanity Fair*, September 2010: 1–5.

Hoffman, Lisa. *The Healing Power of Movement*. New York: Perseus Books Group, 2002.

Holland, Jimmie C., and Sheldon Lewis. *The Human Side of Cancer: Living with Hope, Coping with Uncertainty*. New York: HarperCollins, 2000.

Holmes, Michelle D., Wendy Y. Chen, Diane Feskanich, Candyce H. Kroenke, and Graham A. Colditz. "Physical Activity and Survival after Breast Cancer Diagnosis." *Journal of the American Medical Association* 293, no. 20 (2005): 2479–86.

Holtby, Lisa. *Healing Yoga for People Living with Cancer*. Lanham, MD: Taylor Trade Publishing, 2004.

Iyengar, B. K. S. *Light on Life: The Yoga Journey to Wholeness, Inner Peace, and Ultimate Freedom*. Emmaus, Pa.: Rodale, 2005.

———. *Light on Yoga*. New York: Random House/Schocken Books, 1977.

Johnson, George. *The Cancer Chronicles: Unlocking Medicine's Deepest Mystery*. New York: Alfred A. Knopf, 2013.

Kabat-Zinn, Jon. *Wherever You Go There You Are: Mindfulness Meditation in Everyday Life*. New York: Hyperion, 1994.

Kaelin, Carolyn M., Francesca Coltrea, Josie Gardiner, and Joy Prouty. *The Breast Cancer Survivor's Fitness Plan*. New York: McGraw Hill, 2007.

Kaye, Ronnie. *Spinning Straw into Gold: Your Emotional Recovery from Breast Cancer*. New York: Fireside, 1991.

Khalsa, Sat Bir S., Bethany Butzer, Stephanie M. Shorter, Kristen M. Reinhardt, Stephen Cope. "Yoga Reduces Performance Anxiety in Adolescent Musicians." *Alternative Therapies in Health and Medicine* 19, no. 2 (March/April 2013): 34–45.

Kirkwood, G., H. Rampes, V. Tuffrey, J. Richardson, K. Pilkington. "Yoga for Anxiety: A Systematic Review of the ResearchEvidence" *British Journal of Sports Medicine* 39, no. 12 (December 2005): 884–91. bjsm.bmj.com/content/39/12/884.full.

Kleinberg, Mona. "Working It Out: Exercise and Weight Management for Health and Well-Being." *Insight* (Spring 2006): 1.

Kokkinos, Peter, and Jonathan Myers. "Exercise and Physical Activity; Clinical Outcomes and Applications." *Circulation* 122 (2010): 1637–48. http://circ.ahajournals.org/content/122/16/1637.full.

Kushi, Lawrence H., Colleen Doyle, Marji McCullough, Cheryl L. Rock, Wendy Demark-Wahnefried, Elisa V. Bandera, Susan Gapstur, Alpa V. Patel, Kimberly Andrews, Ted Gansler, and The American Cancer Society 2010 Nutrition and Physical Activity Guidelines Advisory Committee. "American Cancer Society Guidelines on Nutrition and Physical Activity for Cancer Prevention: Reducing the Risk of Cancer with Healthy Food Choices and Physical Activity." *CA: A Cancer Journal for Clinicians* 62 (2012): 30–67, www.onlinelibrary.wiley.com/doi/10.3322/caac.20140/full.

Kytle, Jackson. *To Want to Learn: Insights and Provocations for Engaged Learning.* Second edition. New York: Palgrave Macmillan, 2012.

Langer, Ellen J. *Mindfulness.* Reading, Pa.: Addison-Wesley, 1998.

———. *Counterclockwise: Mindful Health and the Power of Possibility.* New York: Ballantine Books, 2009.

Leaf, Clifton. *The Truth in Small Doses: Why We're Losing the War on Cancer—and How to Win It.* New York: Simon & Schuster, 2013.

Levine, Alison Spatz, and Judith L. Balk. "Yoga and Quality-of-Life Improvement in Patients with Breast Cancer: A Literature Review." *International Journal of Yoga Therapy* 22 (2012): 95–99.

Lewis, Shelly. *Five Lessons I Didn't Learn from Breast Cancer (and One Big One I Did).* New York: Penguin Books, 2008.

Love, Susan. *Dr. Susan Love's Breast Book.* Fifth edition. New York: Da Capo Press, 2010.

Mackenzie, Michael J., Linda E. Carlson, Panteleimon Ekkekakis, David M. Paskevich, and S. Nicole Culos-Reed. "Affect and Mindfulness as Predictors of Change in Mood Disturbance, Stress Symptoms, and Quality of Life in a Community-Based Yoga Program for Cancer Survivors." *Evidence-Based Complementary and Alternative Medicine* (2013): www.ncbi.nlm.nih.gov/pmc/articles/PMC3676912.

Mandal, Ananya. "What Is Gene Expression?" *News Medical* (June 24, 2014): www.news-medical.net/health/What-is-Gene-Expression.aspx.

Mukherjee, Siddhartha. *The Emperor of All Maladies: A Biography of Cancer.* New York: Simon and Schuster, 2011.

Mustian, Karen M., Lisa K. Sprod, Michelle Janelsins, Luke J. Peppone, Oxana G. Palesh, Kavita Chandwani, Pavan S. Reddy, Marianne K. Melnik, Charles Heckler, and Gary R. Morrow. "Multicenter, Randomized Controlled Trial of Yoga for Sleep Quality among Cancer Survivors." *Journal of Clinical Oncology* 31, no. 26 (2013): 3233–41.

Nirmalananda, Swami. *Yogic Management of Cancer*. Bihar, India: Yoga Publications Trust, 2009.

Novotney, Amy. "Yoga as a Practice Tool." *Monitor on Psych*ology 40, no. 10 (November 2009): 38. www.apa.org/monitor/2009/11/yoga.aspx.

Offit, Paul A. *Do You Believe in Magic: The Sense and Nonsense of Alternative Medicine*. New York: Harper, 2013.

Ornish, Dean. *Dr. Dean Ornish's Program for Reversing Heart Disease: The Only System Scientifically Proven to Reverse Heart Disease Without Drugs or Surgery*. New York: Ivy Books, 1996.

———. *The Spectrum: A Scientifically Proven Program to Feel Better, Live Longer, Lose Weight, and Gain Health*. New York: Ballantine, 2007.

Qu, Su, Solveig Mjelstad Olafsrud, Leonardo A. Meza-Zepeda, and Fahri Saatcioglu. "Rapid Gene Expression Changes in Peripheral Blood Lymphocytes upon Practice of a Comprehensive Yoga Program." PLOS ONE (April 17, 2013). DOI: 10.1371/journal.pone.0061910.

Rama, Swami. *Meditation and Its Practice*. Honesdale, Pa.: Himilayan Institute Press, 1992.

Remen, Rachel Naomi. *Kitchen Table Wisdom*. Tenth anniversary edition. New York: Penguin Books, 2006.

Rockhill, Beverly, Walter C. Willett, JoAnn E. Manson, Michael F. Leitzmann, Meir J. Stampfer, David J. Hunter, and Graham A. Colditz. "Physical Activity and Mortality: A Prospective Study Among Women." *American Journal of Public Health* 91, no. 4 (2001): 578–83. www.ncbi.nlm.nih.gov/pmc/articles/PMC1446638/pdf/11291369.pdf.

Rollin, Betty. *Here's the Bright Side: Of Failure, Fear, Cancer, Divorce, and Other Bum Raps*. New York: Random House, 2007.

Satin, Jillian R., Wolfgang Linden, and Roanne D. Millman, "Yoga and Psychophysiological Determinants of Cardiovascular Health: Comparing Yoga Practitioners, Runners, and Sedentary Individuals." *Annals of Behavioral Medicine* 47, no. 2 (2014): 231–41.

Servan-Schreiber, David. *Anticancer: A New Way of Life*. New York: Viking, 2009.

Schaffer, Amanda. "Do Our Bones Influence Our Minds?" *The New Yorker*, November 4, 2013: www.newyorker.com/online/blogs/elements/2013/11/do-our-bones-influence-our-minds.html?printable=true&currentPage=all.

Schnipper, Hester Hill. *After Breast Cancer: A Common-Sense Guide to Life After Treatment*. New York: Bantam Dell, 2006.

Sephton, S. E., F. S. Dhabhar, A. S. Keuroghlian, J. Giese-Davis, B. S. McEwen, A. C. Ionan, and D. Spiegel. "Depression, Cortisol, and Suppressed Cell-mediated Immunity in Metastatic Breast Cancer." *Brain Behavior and Immunity* 23, no. 8 (2009): 1148–55.

Sharma, Manoj, and Taj Haider. "Yoga as an Alternative and Complementary Treatment for Cancer: A Systematic Review." *The Journal of Alternative and Complementary Medicine* 19, no. 11 (2013): 870–75.

Sherman, Paulette Kouffman. *The Cancer Path: A Spiritual Journey into Healing, Wholeness & Love*. New York: Parachute Jump Publishing, 2013. http://parachute-jumppublishing.com.

Silver, Julie K. *After Cancer Treatment: Heal Faster, Better, Stronger*. Baltimore, Md.: The Johns Hopkins University Press, 2006.

Singh, Amika, Léonie Uijtdewilligen, Jos W. R. Twisk, Willem van Mechelen, and Mai J. M. Chinapaw. "Physical Activity and Performance at School: A Systematic Review of the Literature Including a Methodological Quality Assessment." *Archives of Pediatrics and Adolescent Medicine* 166, no. 1 (2012): 49–55. http://archpedi.jamanetwork.com/article.aspx?articleid=1107683.

Smith, Eva Norlyk, and Anita Boser. "Yoga, Vertebral Fractures, and Osteoporosis: Research and Recommendations." *International Journal of Yoga Therapy* 23, no. 1 (2013): 17–23. www.undulationexercise.com/publications/yoga-vertebral-fractures-and-osteoporosis.pdf.

Sontag, Susan. *Illness as Metaphor*. New York: Farrar, Straus and Giroux, 1978.

Sparrowe, Linda and Patricia Walden. *The Woman's Book of Yoga & Health: A Lifelong Guide to Wellness*. Boston: Shambhala Publications, 2002.

Spiegel, David, "Mind Matters in Cancer Survival." *Journal of the American Medical Association* 305, no. 5 (2011): 502–3.

Streeter, Chris C., Theodore H. Whitefield, Liz Owen, Tasha Rein, Surya K. Karri, Aleksandra Yakhkind, Ruth Perlmutter et al., "Effects of Yoga Versus Walking on Mood, Anxiety, and Brain GABA Levels: A Randomized Controlled MRS Study." *The Journal of Alternative and Complementary Medicine* 6, no. 11 (2010): 1145–52. online.liebertpub.com/doi/pdf/10.1089/acm.2010.0007.

Trevino, Haven. *The Tao of Healing: Meditations for Body and Spirit*. Novato, Calif.: New World Library, 1999.

Weed, Susun S. *Breast Cancer? Breast Health!: The Wise Woman Way*. New York: Ash Tree Publishing, 1996.

Weiss, Marisa C. *Living Beyond Breast Cancer: A Survivor's Guide for When Treatment Ends and the Rest of Your Life Begins*. New York: Random House, 1996.

Wilber, Ken. *Grace and Grit: Spirituality and Healing in the Life and Death of Treya Killam Wilber*. Boston: Shambhala Publications, 2001.

"Yoga in America Study 2012." Harris Interactive Service Burreau. www.yogajournal.com/press/yoga_in_america.

Yung, P. S., Y. M. Lai, P. Y. Tung, H. T. Tsui, C. K. Wong, V. W. Hung, and L. Qin. "Effects of Weight Bearing and Non-Weight Bearing Exercises on Bone Properties Using Calcaneal Quantitative Ultrasound." *British Journal of Sports Medicine* 39, no. 8 (2005): 547–51. bjsm.bmj.com/content/39/8/547.long.

Zahavich, Ashley N. Ross, John A. Robinson, David Paskevich, and S. Nicole Culos-Reed. "Examining a Therapeutic Yoga Program for Prostate Cancer Survivors." *Integrative Cancer Therapies* 12, no. 2 (March 2013): 113–25.

Index

BOOKS OF RELATED INTEREST

The Therapeutic Yoga Kit
Sixteen Postures for Self-Healing through Quiet Yin Awareness
by Cheri Clampett and Biff Mithoefer

The Yin Yoga Kit
The Practice of Quiet Power
by Biff Mithoefer

The Heart of Yoga
Developing a Personal Practice
by T. K. V. Desikachar

Natural Posture for Pain-Free Living
The Practice of Mindful Alignment
by Kathleen Porter

Fighting Cancer with Vitamins and Antioxidants
by Kedar N. Prasad, Ph.D., and K. Che Prasad, M.S., M.D.

Delta Medicine
Natural Therapies for the Five Functions of Cellular Health
by Yann Rougier, M.D.

The Healing Intelligence of Essential Oils
The Science of Advanced Aromatherapy
by Kurt Schnaubelt, Ph.D.

Herbs for Healthy Aging
Natural Prescriptions for Vibrant Health
by David Hoffmann, FNIMH, AHG

INNER TRADITIONS • BEAR & COMPANY
P.O. Box 388
Rochester, VT 05767
1-800-246-8648
www.InnerTraditions.com
Or contact your local bookseller

DATE			

Prinster, Tari, 1944- author.
Yoga for cancer.